The Navy SEAL Nutrition Guide

Patricia A. Deuster, Ph.D.
Anita Singh, Ph.D.
Pierre A. Pelletier, ENS, MC, USNR

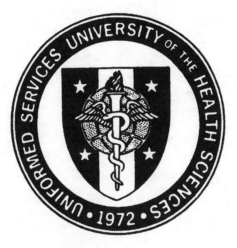

Department of Military and Emergency Medicine
Uniformed Services University of the Health Sciences
F. Edward Hébert School of Medicine

December 1994

Preface

*T*he demands imposed by SEAL training are profound, and success requires the mustering of all your strength - physical and mental. One factor that may bring you closer to success is nutritional interventions. It is well known that appropriate nutritional habits and interventions can enhance your ability to perform, and we want you to be familiar with those successful habits. This manual is for you to read, participate in, and use as a resource when you have questions about nutrition and no one is available to get answers from.

The first five chapters are very basic - they provide background information about nutrition concepts in general, and little to nothing about performance. However, they are very important for fully understanding the information in subsequent chapters. In the remaining chapters, we have tried to be as specific as possible in terms of what we think you should and shouldn't do, and given you reasons for our recommendations. For example, in Chapter 8: Restaurants, Fast Foods, and Eating Out, we have given you sample menus at Fast Foods places so you can select a high carbohydrate diet. In the chapter on Mission Recovery, we target three areas you need to focus on and provide ways to ensure a rapid recovery. In Chapter 15, Ergogenic Agents, we discourage the use of some products because not only is there insufficient information, but there may be potential risks and adverse effects associated with using them. Again, our objective is to make you more informed so you can make educated choices about foods and supplements. Many commercial products sold in stores and through magazines make claims so you will purchase them. With some products you are wasting your money, and with others, possibly hurting yourself. Other products may actually give you the "edge" and improve your performance, but it takes information to make the appropriate decision. This manual should help you do that.

You men are a select group - we know that from our years of working with SEALs and SEAL trainees. For that reason you must be treated as such. This manual has been prepared with that in mind: we want to help you perform to the best of your abilities under the rigorous conditions you confront in training and during missions. We certainly don't have all the answers to nutritional enhancement of performance, because the

---

answers are not all available yet. However, we will continue searching for answers and encourage you to continue asking questions that relate to nutrition and performance so we can help you find those answers. We wish you the best and hope you will let us know when you can't find answers to your questions.

Patty Deuster, Anita Singh, and Pierre Pelletier
Bethesda, MD

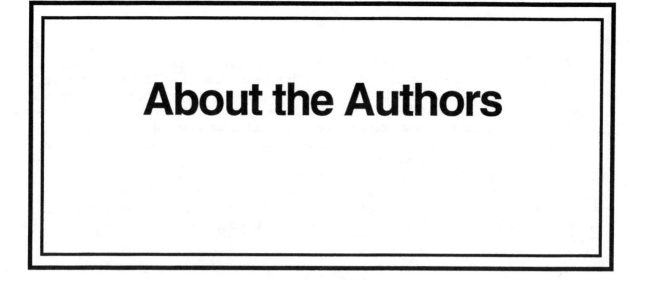

About the Authors

$Dr.$ Patricia Deuster is an Associate Professor and Director of the Human Performance Laboratory in the Department of Military and Emergency Medicine at the Uniformed Services University of the Health Sciences, School of Medicine in Bethesda, Maryland. Her credentials for writing this book are many. She has been conducting research in the area of sports nutrition and exercise physiology for over 14 years, has published numerous papers on the nutritional needs of U.S. Navy SEALs, and has given many sports nutrition seminars to high school, college, and professional athletes, recreational athletes, SWAT teams, dietitians, and other health professionals. She is also an athlete herself. She was a tennis professional for 5 years and has competed in several triathlons and over 20 marathons; her best marathon time was a 2:48 in the Boston Marathon. Dr. Deuster was a nationally ranked runner for several years and a qualifier for the First Women's Olympic Marathon Trials. She is an avid sportswoman and a former skydiver who has logged in over 100 jumps. Together with her athletic abilities and interests, professional training, and research endeavors, she is clearly one of the few persons to have been prepared to develop this guide.

$Dr.$ Anita Singh received her Ph.D. in Nutrition in 1986 from the University of Maryland, where she was selected as an Outstanding Graduate. She is an Assistant Professor in the Department of Military and Emergency Medicine at the Uniformed Services University of the Health Sciences, in Bethesda Maryland. She is also a registered dietitian and has been working in the area of Sports Nutrition for about 10 years. In addition to looking at nutritional needs of U.S. Navy SEAL trainees, she has studied women who qualified for the First Women's Olympic Marathon Trials, triathletes, ultramarathoners and recreational athletes. Dr. Singh has presented her research work at various national and international meetings and has published extensively in scientific journals. She is a runner, tennis player and avid hiker.

*P*ierre A. Pelletier ENS, MC, USNR will be graduating in1995 from the Uniformed Services University of the Health Sciences (USUHS), School of Medicine, in Bethesda, MD. He received his undergraduate degree from Norwich University in Biology and Chemistry. ENS Pelletier has always been active in athletics both as a participant and teacher. He was a competitive skier and instructor for eight years and instructed kayaking in New England. He is also active in the Potomac Rugby Union in Maryland and most recently was invited to play with the US Navy Rugby Club. His personal interest in nutrition as it relates to athletics has been nurtured while at USUHS and culminated in a clinical year of research in the Human Performance Laboratory at USUHS where he assisted in writing the manual. He plans to practice Operational Medicine as a Diving Medical Officer with the US Navy SEALs.

Table of Contents

List of Tables

List of Worksheets

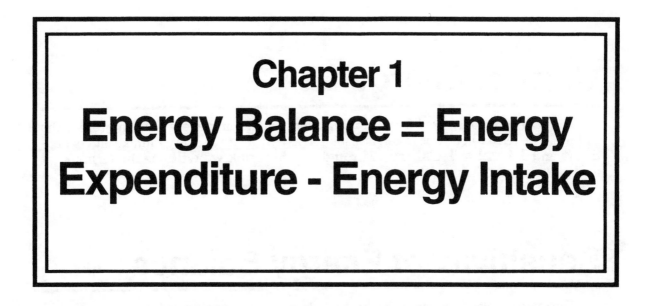

Chapter 1
Energy Balance = Energy Expenditure - Energy Intake

*B*alancing energy intake and expenditure can be difficult when activity levels are very high, as in SEAL training, and when activity levels are very low, such as during isolation. Typically, body weight remains constant when energy intake equals expenditure.

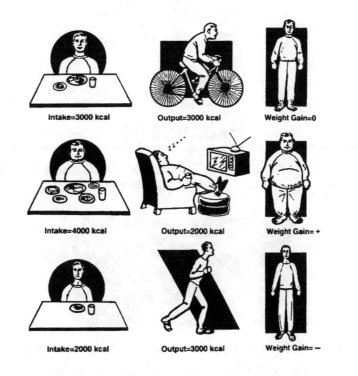

Intake=3000 kcal   Output=3000 kcal   Weight Gain=0

Intake=4000 kcal   Output=2000 kcal   Weight Gain= +

Intake=2000 kcal   Output=3000 kcal   Weight Gain= —

Units of Energy

The unit commonly used for describing energy intake and energy expenditure is the Calorie. The term Kilocalorie (Kcal) is also used as a measure of energy intake and expenditure and **1 Kcal = 1 Calorie. Throughout this book we will use the terms Kcal and calorie interchangeably.**

Sensitivity of Energy Balance

The energy balance equation can be "unbalanced" by changing energy intake, energy expenditure, or both. To gain or lose 1 pound it takes approximately 3500 extra kcal consumed or burned. Believe it or not, the energy balance equation is very sensitive, as is shown in the following example.

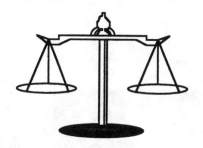

Example 1:

If you ate one extra chocolate chip cookie (65 kcal) each day for one year, this would be 65 X 365 or 23,725 extra kcal.

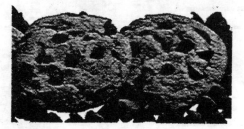

This small daily increase in energy intake would result in a gain of ~ 6.8 pounds in one year.

Energy Balance = Energy Expenditure - Energy Intake

Example 2:

If you ate one less chocolate chip cookie per day and started running 1 extra mile per day 5 days per week, you would lose 14 pounds. This number is obtained by adding the 6.8 pounds from not eating the cookie and the 7.4 pounds/year for running (100 kcal/mile X 5 miles/week X 52 weeks/year = 26,000 kcal or 7.4 pounds/year). **You see? It works both ways!**

Components of Energy Expenditure

The three major contributors to energy expenditure are:

◆ Resting energy expenditure

◆ Physical activity

◆ Energy for digesting foods

The first two are of interest here and will be discussed in detail.

Resting Energy Expenditure

Resting energy expenditure (**REE**) is the amount of energy required to maintain life - such as breathing, beating of the heart, maintenance of body temperature, and other life processes. Measurements are usually made in the morning after waking with the body at complete rest. REE can be estimated by a formula and used to predict your daily energy/ caloric requirements. The only information needed is your body weight in pounds.

Table 1-1. Determining Resting Energy Expenditure (REE) of Men From Body Weight (in pounds)

Age (years)	Equation to Derive REE (kcal/day)
18 - 30	6.95 X Weight + 679
30 - 60	5.27 X Weight + 879

Energy Expenditure For Physical Activity

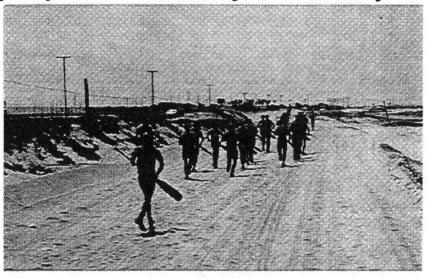

The amount of energy you expend during physical activity is different each day, depending on your training. Some days are very strenuous and involve running, swimming, calisthenics, cold water exposure, sleep deprivation, and carrying heavy loads. Some days you are in the classroom sitting a good portion of the day. Thus, determining your actual energy expended during activity is more difficult, but there are ways to estimate it. You would usually take your REE and multiply it by a number (or factor) as shown on the next page to get a rough estimate of your total energy/calorie needs. Lets try out an example.

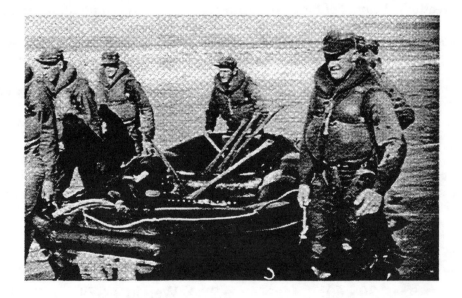

Total Energy Expenditure

Table 1-2. Estimating Total Daily Energy Needs of Men at Various Levels of Activity

Level of General Activity	Activity Factor (X REE)
Very Light - Seated and standing activities, driving, playing cards	1.3
Light - walking, carpentry, sailing, playing ping- pong or pool, golf	1.6
Moderate - carrying a load, jogging, light swimming, biking, calisthenics, scuba diving	1.7
Heavy - walking with a load uphill, rowing, digging, climbing, soccer, basketball, running, obstacle course	2.1
Exceptional - running/ swimming races, cycling uphill, carrying very heavy loads, hard rowing	2.4

Example: You are 21, weigh 175 lbs, and activity is moderate

REE = 6.95 X Weight + 679 = 6.95 X 175 + 679 = 1895 kcal/day

Total Energy Needs = 1895 X 1.7 = 3222 kcal/day

The formula for REE came from Table 1-1.

The 1.7 is the Activity Factor for "Moderate" from the table above.

Worksheet 1-1. Estimate Your Total Daily Energy Needs

Weight: _195_ Age: _19_ Activity Factor: _2.1_

Determine Your REE: _~~2000~~ 2034_ kcal/day

Energy Needs = REE X Activity = _2034_ X _2.1_

My Estimated Energy Needs = _4272_ kcal/day

Body Size and Body Mass Index

The BODY MASS INDEX, or BMI is a measure commonly used to rapidly assess body composition and then classify and identify individuals as under-, overweight or overfat. The BMI is actually a ratio: weight/height^2, with weight in kilograms and height in meters. Reference standards have been developed for the United States population as a whole, broken down by race and gender, so that individuals at risk for obesity can be identified. However, the reference values for the U.S. population as a whole do not always apply to special populations, such as SEALs. As a result, unique populations often develop their own standards and references based on individuals within that population. A reference range based on a survey of over 800 SEALs was recently developed. For all the SEALs combined, the average BMI was 25, and the average body fat was 13%. What is important to remember, is that this index is a screening tool. You can use the BMI to assess and keep track of changes in your body composition. If your BMI is high, have your body fat checked, and if your body fat is more than 20%, you need to take some action to lower your weight. Reference BMI values for you are provided below:

Reference BMI Values for SEALs	
Lean	<20
Typical SEAL	20 to 29
Check Your Body Fat	29 to 32

Use the nomogram below to find your BMI and see where you fall relative to the reference values. To use the nomogram, place a ruler or straight edge between height (right side) and body weight (left side); then read BMI from the central scale. **NOTE:** Even with these reference values, the BMI can misclassify some large frame, very strong men as overweight. Check your body fat; that will be the deciding factor.

Worksheet 1-2. Normogram for Body Mass Index

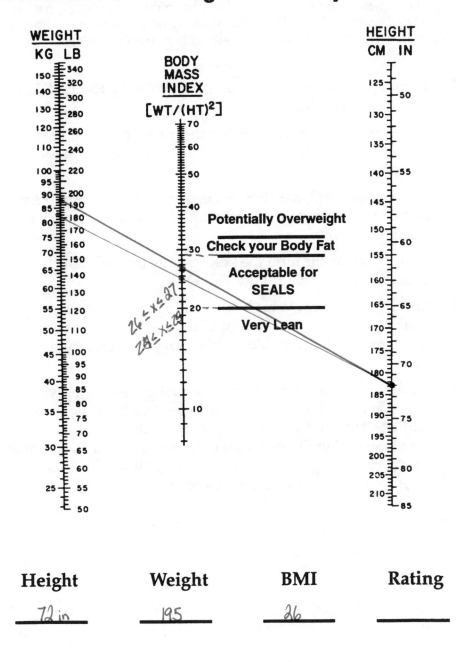

Height	Weight	BMI	Rating
72 in	195	26	

How To Calculate Energy Expenditure

You will need a calculator to complete this exercise.

Over a 24 hour period you will expend different amounts of energy in each activity in which you engage, be it watching TV, eating, running on the sand, paddling, or listening to your teammates. The objective of this activity is to make you aware of the energy you actually do expend.

♦ Record your name and date on your **ENERGY EXPENDITURE ACTIVITY FORM**.

♦ List all the activities you participated in over the last 12 hours and the approximate length of time (in minutes) you spent on each activity on the form.

♦ Go through the alphabetical list of activities provided in **Appendix 4**, and find the activity that most closely approximates each one you listed on the form.

♦ Write down on the form the kcal/minute (not per hour!) value in the appropriate column (**Energy Value**).

♦ Multiply the energy value by the total time in minutes. For example, if you ran in the sand in boots for 25 minutes, then your energy expenditure for that activity would be 15 (energy value) X 25 (time) = 385 kcals.

♦ Do this for at least five activities, or preferably all the events in 12 hours. Then add up the numbers to get an actual energy expenditure estimate. How did you fare? You were probably surprised by some of the numbers, but this experience should give you a good overview of energy balance. Keep track of your weight if you are in doubt - it is the most accurate way to monitor energy balance.

Worksheet 1-3. Energy Expenditure Activity Form

Name: Daniel Horn   **Date:** 6/8/04

Activity	Time in Minutes	Energy Value (kcal/min)	Total Calories
Obstacle Course	30	10	300
4 mile run, 8 min/mile pace	32	14	448
5 Mile Ocean Swim	175	9	1575
Calisthenics	30	8	240
Weight Lifting	45	11	495
14 Mile Run in boots	140	12	1680
5 Mile Hike w/80 lb load	100	14	1400
Class	195 min	2	390
Walking	60 min	9	540
Weightlifting	45 min	11	495
Sitting at ease	120 min	1	120
Running -	35 min	17	595
Swimming -	40 min	11	440
Pushups	3 min	6	18
Situps	3 min	5	15
~~Walking~~ Sleeping	51 min	2	102
GRAND TOTAL			2715

Chapter 2
Carbohydrate, Fat and Protein: The Energy-Providing Macronutrients

*Y*ou have heard the saying *"You are what you eat"*. Although this statement has not been proven, we do know that what you eat makes a difference in how you perform, how long you survive, and the quality of your life. The *macronutrients*, or energy-providing nutrients, are extremely important in this respect. Also, without energy you would starve, and your ability to perform would be greatly reduced. Our three main sources of energy are:

◆ Carbohydrate or **CHO**

◆ Fat

◆ Protein

These fuels are called *macro* because they are eaten in "large quantities" unlike the micronutrients we will discuss later. This chapter will provide basic information about these *macronutrients*.

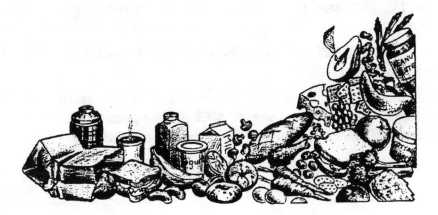

Carbohydrate

Carbohydrates, commonly abbreviated CHO, are foods we want to become very familiar with since they are the preferred foods for endurance activities, competitive athletic events, and healthy living. In fact, CHOs are the basic source of energy for humans. Luckily, CHO are also foods you are encouraged to eat, not foods you are urged to restrict, such as fat.

Definition, Composition, and Classification

Carbohydrates are composed of three elements: carbon, hydrogen and oxygen. They exist in many forms, but the two major types of CHOs are simple and complex.

- Simple CHOs have one (mono) or two (disaccharides) sugar molecules hooked together.

- Types of simple CHOs include glucose (dextrose), table sugar (sucrose), honey (fructose and glucose), fructose (sugars in fruit), maltose (sugars in malt), lactose (sugar in milk), brown sugar, corn syrup, maple syrup, refined sugar products, raw sugar, corn sweeteners, high-fructose corn syrup, and molasses.

- Complex CHOs have three or more simple sugar molecules hooked together; polysaccharides are long strands of simple sugars.

- Complex CHOs are found in grains, fruits, seeds, potatoes, pasta, macaroni, seaweed, algae, and legumes such as peas and beans, and all other vegetables.

- The main forms of complex CHOs are starches and fibers; they come from plant materials. Starches are digested by the body whereas dietary fiber cannot be. Fiber will be discussed in Chapter 5.

- The only CHO stored in animals is "glycogen" which is found in liver and muscles.

- The amount of glycogen stored in liver and muscle is limited: muscle glycogen stores can be depleted after 3 to 4 hours of heavy exercise and a 24 hour fast could use up liver glycogen stores.

Functions of Carbohydrate in the Body

CHOs are used in the body mainly as:

- *Fuel in the form of glucose* - glucose is the most important source of energy in our body, and it is stored in the liver and muscle as glycogen. The complex CHOs you eat are digested into simple sugars, mostly glucose, and then used by the muscles, brain, heart, and other organs for energy.

- Building blocks to make chemicals needed by the cells of your body

- Chemical cement for repairing structures of your body

Carbohydrate in the Diet

CHO foodstuffs are the largest part of the world's food supply. In Mexico the CHO staples are corn tortilla and beans; in Brazil - black beans and rice; in India - chick peas (garbanzo), lentils, rice, and whole grain unleavened breads; in Japan - rice, tofu and vegetables; and in the Middle East - humus (chick peas) and tahini (sesame seeds). In the United States our classic CHOs are bread, potatoes, noodles, and macaroni.

Unfortunately, many people think starches are unhealthy and lead to weight gain. That notion came about because most people add high fat toppings and/or sauces to their starchy foods. For example, many individuals put lots of butter or margarine on their bread, sour cream on their baked potato, cream cheese on bagels and cream sauces on their macaroni or pasta! Look below to see what kinds of foods provide simple and complex CHOs.

Energy From Carbohydrate

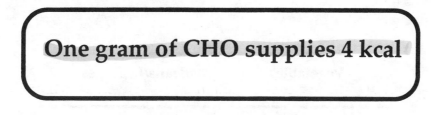

One gram of CHO supplies 4 kcal

EXAMPLE: One Fig Newton contains 10 grams of CHO and provides 60 calories. Calories from CHO and percent of calories from CHO are:

$$4 \text{ kcal} \times 10 \text{ grams} = 40 \text{ kcal from CHO}$$

$$40/60 = 0.67 = 67\% \text{ of energy from CHO}$$

Table 2-1. Ideas For Selecting Foods/ Food Combinations High In Complex CHO

Below are some suggestions for foods to eat at meal and snack times. Fruits are always good - especially since they also provide water which is very important.

Breakfast Cereals	Grains	Fruits
Oatmeal	Bagel with Jam	Oranges
Wheaties	Whole Wheat Bread	Banana
Cornflakes	English Muffin	Cantaloupe
Wheatena	Pancakes	Peaches
Cheerios	Rice	Apples
Raisin Bran	White Potatoes	Pineapple
Grapenuts	Sweet Potatoes	Grapefruit
Granola	Macaroni/Noodles	Strawberries
	Tortilla	
	Waffles	
	Muffins, bran, blueberry etc	

Vegetables	Beans/Legumes
Tomato/Tomato Sauce	Kidney Beans
Carrots and Peas	Lentil Stew
Eggplant	Chick-peas

Vegetables	Beans/Legumes
Squash	Black-eyed Peas
Broccoli	Lima Beans
Cauliflower	Pinto Beans

Sandwiches and Fillings	Other Ideas

Sandwiches and Fillings	Other Ideas
French Roll w/ Tuna, Lettuce, Pickles	Pasta with Turkey and Veggies
Pita w/ Turkey, Lettuce, Mustard	Rice with Chicken and Veggies
Chicken, Lettuce, Mustard on Rye	Pasta with Tuna, Celery, Onions
Bagel with Peanut Butter and Jelly	Fruit Salad
Pita w/ Mashed Beans, Onions	Spaghetti and Sauce
Tortilla with Beans, Lettuce	Chicken Noodle Soup
Chicken Burrito	Potato Salad

Low Fat/High CHO	High Fat/High CHO
Any Kind of Fruit	Most Cookies
Raisins, Dates, Prunes	Most Cakes
Popcorn, Pretzels	Candy Bars
Bagel with Jam	Ice Creams

Fat

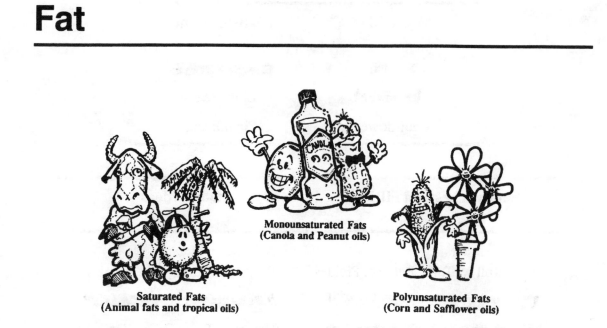

Monounsaturated Fats
(Canola and Peanut oils)

Saturated Fats
(Animal fats and tropical oils)

Polyunsaturated Fats
(Corn and Safflower oils)

Believe it or not, fat is an essential part of your diet, even though you hear everyone say "Don't eat that, it's high in fat!". Fat adds taste to foods and satisfies your sense of hunger. However, not all fats are created equal. By understanding the different types of dietary fat, how fat works in the body, and using guidelines for daily fat consumption, you can eliminate excess fat from your diet and eat for better health.

Definition, Composition, and Classification

Fat is an essential nutrient for your body, and is usually classified according to its chemical form. There are three major types of fats or fatty acids:

◆ Saturated

◆ Monounsaturated

◆ Polyunsaturated

Saturated fats ("fatty acids") which are solid at room temperature, have no room for any additional hydrogen atoms. Saturated fats are found primarily in animal foods—red meats, lard, butter, poultry with skin, and whole milk dairy products. Palm, palm kernel and coconut oils are also highly saturated.

Mono and polyunsaturated fats, which remain liquid at room temperature have room for additional hydrogen atoms. Monounsaturates have room for only one hydrogen and are found in olives, olive oil, avocados, and peanuts. Polyunsaturated fats, which have room for more than one hydrogen, are found primarily in fish, corn, wheat, nuts, seeds, and vegetable oils, such as peanut, sunflower, corn and safflower oils.

Functions of Fat in the Body

Fats, or fatty acids, serve several important roles in the body. Fat:

◆ Is our major form of stored energy; it provides energy during exercise, in cold environments, and when you don't have enough to eat

◆ Insulates the body

◆ Helps carry other nutrients to places in the body

◆ Protects organs

◆ Serves a structural role in cells

Despite its bad reputation, fat is very important, and some fats/fatty acids are essential.

How Much Fat Should We Eat?

A little of all the different types of fats is desirable, but **TOO** much fat is the primary dietary problem in our country. A high intake of fat is associated with many diseases, including:

◆ Heart disease   ◆ Many forms of cancer

◆ Obesity   ◆ Diabetes

The average American consumes 42% of his or her daily calories as fat (40% carbohydrate and 18% protein). **Most health experts agree that Americans should decrease their fat intake to no more than 30% of the total daily calories, and saturated fat should provide no more than 10% of the total daily calories.** In our country, more than 15% of our calories are from saturated fat. The key to this is knowing which foods are high in fat and which are low. Once you have that information, it is up to you to start changing your dietary behaviors.

Energy From Fat

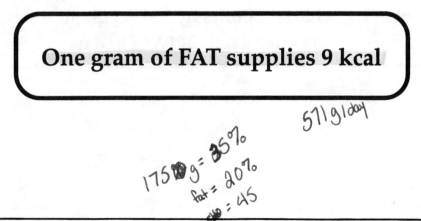

One gram of FAT supplies 9 kcal

571 g/day

1750 g = 35%
fat = 20%
= 45

Fat provides more than twice the energy supplied by carbohydrates.

Example 1:

A 1 ounce bag of potato chips contains 10 grams of fat, so the calories from fat are:

9 kcal X 10 grams = 90 kcal of energy

Example 2:

One hot dog supplies17 grams of fat, so calories from fat would be:

9 kcal X 17 grams = 153 kcal of energy

Determining Your Daily Fat Allowance

Everyone talks about grams of fat, but what does that mean on a practical level? How does one translate "grams" of fat to percent fat and how many grams of fat should you allow yourself each day? You know that only 30% of your calories should come from fat, so with that in mind, you will learn how to determine your daily fat allowance. Let's take an example first:

Example: Determining A Fat Allowance

If estimated energy need (EEN)= 3222 calories

Step 1. Multiply EEN by 0.3 to get calories from fat
3222 X 0.3 = 967 fat calories

Step 2. Divide fat calories by 9 to get grams of fat.
967/9 = 107 grams of FAT per day

Where Did the Numbers Come From?

◆ Estimated energy need was provided in the example. You know your EEN from the previous chapter.

◆ **0.3** in Step 1 is for calculating 30% of calories from fat.

◆ **9** in Step 2 is the number of calories in one gram of fat.

◆ **107** is the number of grams of fat that should not be exceeded to ensure that the diet provides no more than 30% of calories from fat.

Worksheet 2-1. Figure Out Your Fat Allowance

Refer back to your Estimated energy needs (EEN) exercise (Chapter 1, page 6) and write your EEN in the box below.

Estimated Energy Need (EEN) =

STEP 1. EEN X 0.3 = ~~4005~~ 4272 **X 0.3**

Calories from Fat = ~~811005~~ 1281.6

STEP 2. Calories from Fat/9 = ~~8005~~ 1281.6 **/9**

Grams of Fat per Day = ~~9005~~ 142.4

Now that you know how to do this, just take whatever percent fat you want, multiply it by your energy needs, and then divide by 9.

You can also use the above method to determine the percent of fat in particular foods. If you read a food label and it shows the item provides 270 calories, of which 15 grams are fat, then to calculate the percent of calories from fat you would do the following:

Total Calories = 270

Total Fat = 15 grams

Calories from Fat = 15 grams X 9 kcal = 135 kcal

% Calories from Fat = (135 X 100)/270 = 50%

Worksheet 2-2. Calculating Percent of Calories From Fat

Food	Total Calories	Grams of Fat	Fat Calories	% of Calories
Hot Dog	183	16.6	16.6 X 9 = 149.4	149 X 100/183 = 81.6%
Double Cheese Pizza, 1 slice	370	19	19 X 9 = 171	171 X 100/370 = 46.2%
Barbecue Potato Chips	278	18.4	18.4 X 9 = 166	166 X 100/278 = 59.7%
Tootsie Roll	112	2.5		
BLT Sandwich w/ Mayo	282	15.6		

Worksheet 2-3. Select A "Lower Fat" Alternative

Below is a list of foods that are high in fat. Look at each food item and determine a suitable replacement that you think would be much lower in fat.

FOOD	REPLACEMENT
French Fries with Ketchup	Boiled Potatoes
Chicken Drumstick w/ Skin	Chicken Breast w/o Skin
Beef Hot Dog	Chicken or Turkey Dog
Tuna Packed in Oil	Tuna Packed in Water
Whole Milk	Skim or 1% Milk
Regular Cottage Cheese	1% Fat Cottage Cheese
Regular Ice Cream	Ice Milk or Italian Ice
Ground Beef	Ground Turkey or Extra Lean Beef
Baked Potato and Sour Cream	Baked Potato with Yogurt
Bagel with Cream Cheese	
Whole Milk Yogurt	

FOOD	REPLACEMENT
Cheese Sandwich	
Turkey Sandwich with Mayonnaise	
Pizza with Double Cheese	
Salad with Blue Cheese Dressing	
Potato Chips with Dip	
Bologna and Cheese Sandwich	

Protein

Many people like to eat high protein foods because they think protein makes them grow "big and strong". Are they correct? Let's take a look at protein and what it really does.

Definition and Composition

Unlike carbohydrates and fats which contain only carbon, oxygen and hydrogen, protein also contains *nitrogen* and other elements essential for life. Proteins are made up of several *amino acids* - small building blocks that are hooked together. Although there are many different amino acids (at least 20), only 9 are called *essential amino acids* because the body cannot make them; they must be obtained from the diet. That's why we must eat protein - to take in the essential amino acids.

Functions of Protein in the Body

Proteins vary in size, depending on how many amino acids are linked together, and each one performs different functions in the body. Although they can provide energy, they are not a main source of energy like carbohydrates and fat. Some functions of protein are:

◆ Form muscle, hair, nails, skin, and other tissues

◆ Direct energy production

◆ Repair injuries

◆ Carry fats, vitamins and minerals to different parts of the body

◆ Muscle contraction

◆ Serve a structural role for every part of the body

How Much Protein Should I Eat?

Many people eat 150 to 200 g of protein each day which is more protein than is actually needed by the body. Protein needs are determined by age, body weight, and activity level. Many athletes think that if they eat more protein their muscles will get larger, but this is not true. Excess calories from protein can be converted to fat and stored. Additionally, the liver and the kidneys are put under a lot of strain when processing large quantities of protein.

Table 2-2. How Much Protein Do I Need?

Grams of Protein Per Pound of Body Weight

Activity Level	Protein Factor
Low to Moderate	0.5 grams
Endurance Training	0.6 - 0.8 grams
Strength/Weight Training	0.6 - 0.8 grams

Example

Suppose you weigh 175 pounds and are training to be a SEAL. Then you are "IN TRAINING" for sure - both endurance and strength training. Your protein needs would be 0.6 to 0.8 grams per pound body weight, as shown in the figure above.

Protein Needs = 0.8 X 175 = 140 grams

Worksheet 2-4. Calculate Your Protein Needs

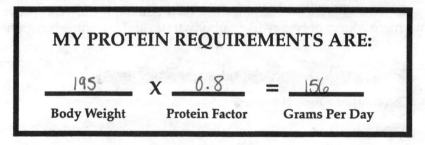

MY PROTEIN REQUIREMENTS ARE:

$$\underset{\text{Body Weight}}{\underline{195}} \quad X \quad \underset{\text{Protein Factor}}{\underline{0.8}} \quad = \quad \underset{\text{Grams Per Day}}{\underline{156}}$$

Energy from Protein

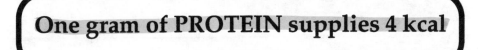

One gram of PROTEIN supplies 4 kcal

Protein supplies about the same energy as carbohydrates.

Example 1:

One hard boiled egg contains 6 grams of protein; calories from protein are:

4 kcal X 6 grams = 24 kcal of energy

Example 2:

One small hamburger supplies 24 grams of protein; calories from protein would be:

4 kcal X 24 grams = 96 kcal of energy

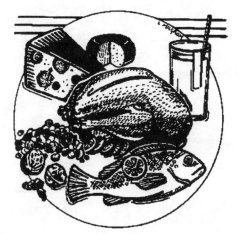

Chapter 3
Micronutrients:
Vitamins and Minerals

Micronutrients are substances required by or essential to the body in very small amounts and include both vitamins and minerals. Taking in either too little or too much of these nutrients can interfere with normal bodily functions. It is difficult to consume excessive amounts through a typical diet. However, it is possible to obtain too little of selected vitamins and minerals if proper food selections are not made.

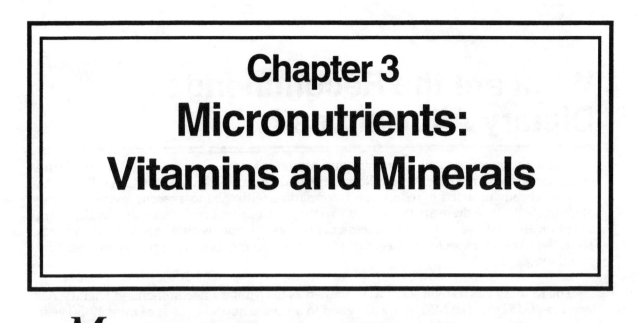

Vitamin E

α-TOCOPHEROL

Vitamin C

ASCORBIC ACID

Pro-Vitamin A

β-CAROTENE

What are the Recommended Dietary Allowances?

The amounts of particular vitamins and minerals a normal person should eat to prevent a deficiency are known as the Recommended Dietary Allowances (RDA). The RDA are periodically updated to reflect new information, with the most recent revision taking place in 1989. Since there are individual variations in nutrient requirements, the RDA are based on the average nutrient requirements of most people with a safety factor added. Thus, the RDA are expected to meet the nutrient requirements of most people in a healthy population.

The Military has its own set of RDA known as the Military Recommended Dietary Allowances (MRDA). The MRDA are designed to meet the nutrient needs of most 17-50 year old moderately active, military personnel. In some cases the allowances are similar but in others the MRDA are slightly higher. This is because the last version of the MRDA was in 1980. Neither the RDA nor the MRDA considers the nutrient needs of special populations, such as SEALs who are extremely active and train and operate under diverse, often gruelling, environmental conditions. Therefore, both sets of recommendations can serve only as guidelines for your minimal intake. In most instances your micronutrient needs will be met through increased food intake provided you eat a variety of foods.

What are Vitamins?

Vitamins are organic compounds that do not provide calories. They are broadly classified into two categories:

- ◆ Fat soluble vitamins
- ◆ Water soluble vitamins

Fat soluble vitamins, which include vitamins A, D, E and K, are absorbed with dietary fat, can be stored in various tissues such as the liver, and are not excreted in the urine. In contrast, water soluble vitamins, which include all B vitamins and vitamin C (ascorbic acid), are not stored in the body in appreciable amounts and small amounts are excreted in the urine each day.

What Functions Do Vitamins Serve?

Vitamins perform a wide variety of functions, including the release of energy from macronutrients (carbohydrate, fat and protein), tissue growth and repair, maintenance and support of reproductive function, and production of an immune response. Some functions may be specific to only one vitamin, whereas some functions may require more than one vitamin. For example, several B vitamins and some minerals are required for releasing energy from macronutrients as shown below.

Table 3-1. Recommended Intakes and Functions of Vitamins

Vitamin	RDA for Men*	Important Functions
Vitamin A (retinol, retinoids)	1000 µg Retinol Equivalents (RE) or 5000 International Units (IU)	Antioxidant. Important for making proteins in tendons and bone. Protects the skin from sun ultraviolet damage. Protects lungs against pollutants. Needed for dark adaptation. May reduce risk of cataracts. Enhances resistance to infections. Supports immune function.
Carotenes: beta carotene converts to vitamin A in healthy people		Water soluble, safe form of vitamin A that is not stored. Same functions as vitamin A. Stronger antioxidant than vitamin A.
Vitamin D	10 µg or 400 IU	Regulates calcium metabolism and bone mineralization.
Vitamin E	10 mg α– Tocopherol Equivalents (TE) or 10 IU	Antioxidant. Protector of cell membranes. Protective against detrimental effects of environmental toxins. Enhances immune function.
Vitamin K	1 µg/kg body weight	Assists in blood clotting. Participates in calcium metabolism.
Vitamin B$_1$ (thiamin)	1.5 mg	Participates in energy production, CHO metabolism, and growth. Supports muscle and cardiovascular function.
Vitamin B$_2$ (riboflavin)	1.7 mg	Energy production from CHO, fat and protein metabolism. Needed for growth and tissue repair.

Table 3-1. Recommended Intakes and Functions of Vitamins

Vitamin	RDA for Men*	Important Functions
Vitamin B$_3$ (niacin, niacinamide, nicotinic acid)	19 mg of Niacin Equivalents (NE)	Energy production from CHO, fat and protein metabolism. Essential for aerobic metabolism.
Vitamin B$_5$ (pantothenic acid)	4 - 7 mg	Essential for energy production from CHO and fat metabolism. Maintains normal growth and function of cells. Needed for proper function and production of anti–stress actions.
Vitamin B$_6$ (pyridoxine HCl, pyridoxal 5'-phosphate)	2 mg	Essential for protein metabolism and immune function. Supports red blood cell production. Promotes healthy skin and connective tissues. Helps prevent and treat repetitive motion injury such as carpal tunnel syndrome. Required to release glucose from CHO stored in muscle as glycogen.
Vitamin B$_{12}$ (cobalamin)	2 µg	Required for red blood cell synthesis. Promotes growth and energy production.
Biotin	30 - 100 µg	Participates in fat and glycogen metabolism.
Folate (folic acid, folacin)	200 µg	Vital for red blood cell synthesis. Essential for the proper division of cells.
Vitamin C (ascorbic acid, ascorbate)	60 mg	Antioxidant. Primary role in growth and repair of connective tissues and bone. Increases resistance to infection and supports optimal immune function. Essential for proper function and production of stress hormones. Accelerates wound healing and repair. Increases resistance to environmental toxins.

* From the 1989 RDA for normal healthy men 19 to 50 years. CHO = carbohydrate.

What Foods are Good Sources of Vitamins?

No one food is a good source of all vitamins and as such a variety of foods should be consumed. Some foods are very high in selected vitamins whereas some contain precursors or substances that serve as building blocks for making the vitamin in the body. For example, beta carotene and other carotenoids from plant foods are converted by an enzyme in the body to vitamin A. Some processed foods provide many vitamins because they have been fortified with nutrients. Other foods will contain few, if any, vitamins. Make sure you READ FOOD LABELS to see how much of the RDA the food contains.

Food preparation techniques can affect the final amount of a particular vitamin in a food; this is specially true when cooking vegetables. Of all vitamins, vitamin C is most easily destroyed during cooking and as such raw fruits and juices are preferred sources of this vitamin. Steps you can take to increase the retention of vitamins while preparing a meal include:

- Avoid soaking vegetables in water
- Cook vegetables in just enough water to prevent burning
- Use the shortest cooking time by cooking vegetables to a crisp and tender stage
- Steaming and stir frying result in the best vitamin retention
- Use leftover cooking water in soups and sauces whenever possible to use the water soluble vitamins that were leached out
- Cut and cook vegetables shortly before serving or refrigerate in an airtight storage container.

If you are not responsible for cooking your meals or if you eat in the galley, the key is to eat a variety of foods when possible. If you are eating field rations during training or deployment, eat the entrees as well as the other food and beverage items provided in the pack. For example, cocoa in the MRE ration is a source of vitamin B_1, calcium and magnesium. Good food sources of the vitamins are provided in Appendix 5.

What are Minerals

Minerals are inorganic compounds found in all body tissues and account for 4 to 5% of a persons total body weight. Typically they are classified as minerals, trace minerals and electrolytes, depending on how much is found in the body and the functions they serve. For example, calcium and magnesium are minerals, whereas zinc, copper and iron are trace minerals, because the body contains small amounts of them. Sodium, potassium and chloride are the primary electrolytes.

What Functions Do Minerals Serve?

Minerals carry "charges", either positive or negative, which help determine their functions. Like vitamins, minerals are essential for a variety of important physiological functions, such as regulation of fluid balance, conduction of nerve impulses, muscle contraction as well as others. Selected functions and the Recommended Dietary Allowances for the most of the essential minerals are presented in the next table.

Table 3-2. Recommended Intakes and Functions of Minerals

Mineral	RDA for Men	Important Functions
Boron	Unknown	Important in bone retention.
Calcium	1200 mg	Essential for growth and structural integrity of bones. Important to nerve conduction and muscle contraction-relaxation.
Chromium[1]	50 - 200 μg	Participates in CHO and fat metabolism. Works with insulin to promote proper glucose utilization. May have an anabolic effect on body composition.
Copper[1]	1.5 - 3 mg	Essential for oxygen-carrying hemoglobin synthesis. Involved in energy production, cardiac function, and regulation of inflammation. Essential for the antioxidant enzyme super oxide dismutase (SOD).
Iron	15 mg	Essential for the production of hemoglobin in red blood cells and myoglobin in skeletal muscle. Essential cofactor for detoxification and energy producing enzyme systems.
Magnesium	350 mg	Essential for nerve impulse conduction and muscle contraction-relaxation. Essential for CHO metabolism. Essential for proper calcium utilization and metabolism.

Mineral	RDA for Men	Important Functions
Manganese[1]	2 - 5 mg	Essential to formation and integrity of connective tissue. Important in normal immune and nervous system function.
Phosphorous	1200 mg	Essential for energy production. Involved in most physicochemical reactions in the body. Integral component to all cell membranes, nerve tissue, and bone. Needed for transfer of nerve impulses. Involved in calcium balance.
Potassium	2000 mg	Essential for nerve impulse conduction. Important for regulating water balance in the body. Important in regulating acid-base balance. Essential for normal heart beat and rhythm.
Selenium	70 µg	Antioxidant. Works with vitamin E to reduce oxidation damage to tissues. Supports proper cardiovascular and immune function.
Sodium[2]	500 - 2,400 mg	Essential for nerve impulse conduction and muscle contraction. Essential for fluid balance and acid-base balance.
Zinc	15 mg	Participates in formation of proteins. Involved in skeletal muscle metabolism. Important for proper neurologic functions. Supports immune function and increases resistance to infections. Enhances wound healing.

[1]Estimated safe and adequate daily intake range - meets requirements of individuals and avoids the danger of toxicity (Food and Nutrition Board, 1989).

[2]The minimum daily requirement for sodium is 500 mg or 1250 mg of salt. Salt is 40% sodium and 60% chloride. 1 teaspoon of salt (sodium chloride) = 5g provides 5 X 40/100 = 2 g of sodium; 2 g is the same as 2000 mg. The minimum daily requirement for potassium is 2000 mg.

What Foods are Good Sources of Minerals?

As with vitamins, a variety of foods should be eaten in order to meet your mineral requirements. The amount of a particular mineral that will be absorbed from foods varies widely and depends upon a number of factors. Absorption of minerals can be influenced by:

◆ Other dietary constituents, such as dietary fiber, oxalates and phytates

- ◆ The amount of other minerals in the diet
- ◆ Medications
- ◆ The body's need for the mineral
- ◆ Chemical form of the mineral
- ◆ Integrity of the intestinal tract

Even though foods may contain certain minerals, other food constituents can influence the actual amount absorbed. For example, insoluble materials like dietary fiber, phytates (chemicals found in high fiber foods) and oxalates (chemicals found in certain foods such as spinach, chard, and rhubarb) bind minerals including iron, calcium and zinc to make them less available for absorption. In contrast, the presence of vitamin C improves the absorption of calcium, iron and zinc. The absorption of iron is dependent on its particular form: heme or non-heme. Heme iron is found in animal foods and is better absorbed than non-heme iron from plant foods. Finally, excessive intakes of some minerals can interfere with the absorption of others: high intakes of supplemental zinc can decrease copper absorption and high iron intakes can decrease zinc absorption. Good food sources of minerals are listed in Appendix 6.

What Substances May Interfere With Micronutrients?

Many things you take or do can affect your losses of vitamins and minerals. In particular, substances that act as "ANTI" vitamins/minerals and may interfere with the amounts of vitamins and minerals in your body include:

Caffeine	**Aspirin**
Tobacco	**Alcohol**
Antibiotics	**Stress**

Summary

The key to meeting your vitamin and mineral needs is eating a diet containing a variety of foods. Remember, food preparation can affect micronutrient content, and that simple changes, such as drinking water or juice instead of tea or coffee with meals can increase absorption of many minerals. If you do not eat alot of fresh fruits and vegetables, then try to eat fortified, ready to eat, breakfast cereals in the morning and for snacks. If you are in doubt about the nutrient content of a processed food, just look at food labels. Most unprocessed foods are nutritious. The following practices will help ensure that you meet your daily vitamin and mineral needs:

Eat A Variety of Foods

Be Savvy in Your Food Selections

Use Good Food Preparation Techniques

Vitamin and mineral supplements are being widely used by physically active people because of all the performance enhancing claims made by supplement manufacturers. It is estimated that about 40 - 50% of athletes use some form of vitamin/mineral supplements. These include single vitamins (such as vitamin C) or minerals (such as iron) and multivitamin-mineral combinations in doses that range from amounts that are similar to the Recommended Dietary Allowances (RDA) up to levels many times the RDA (see Chapter 3 for information on the RDAs).

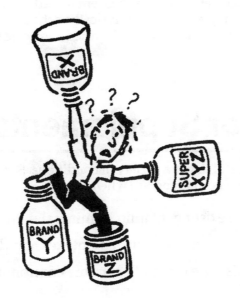

Role of Vitamins and Minerals in Physical Activity

Vitamins and minerals are required in micro (very small, minute) amounts by the body to perform vital metabolic and physiologic functions. Some of the functions related to physical activity that vitamins and minerals are involved in include:

◆ Production of energy: many vitamins and minerals are involved in producing energy from carbohydrates (CHO), fats and proteins.

◆ Formation of red blood cells: some vitamins and minerals are also required for the formation of red blood cells. Red blood cells contain hemoglobin, an iron containing protein that carries oxygen.

◆ Providing oxygen to the exercising muscles: hemoglobin and myoglobin are iron containing proteins which transport and deliver oxygen to exercising muscles.

◆ Maintenance of healthy muscles and joints.

◆ Recovery from exercise: some vitamins and minerals may help in recovering from exhaustive exercise.

Because of all the functions served by vitamins and minerals (see Chapter 3 for additional information), the supplement industry has embarked on a promotional campaign to encourage the use of supplements by physically active people. Whether all the hype about supplement use and performance is justified is discussed below.

Benefits of Supplementation

Supplements are useful under a variety of conditions. Some conditions where benefits of supplementation have been found are when:

◆ There is an existing vitamin or mineral deficiency

◆ Individuals have poor nutrient intakes and dietary habits

◆ Individuals are exposed to extreme environmental conditions, such as altitude

Supplement Use and Performance

Vitamin Supplements

Taking a general multivitamin supplement appears to be without measurable performance enhancing effects in healthy, well-nourished, physically active men on measures of maximal aerobic capacity, heart rate, submaximal endurance running performance, and muscle glycogen stores. Similarly, no improvements in muscle strength or endurance have been noted in strength athletes, such as body builders, who tend to use megadoses of vitamin and mineral supplements.

We don't know yet whether supplementation with various nutrients will have other more subtle beneficial effects that may allow you to perform at an optimal level for extended periods of time. For example, supplementation with selected vitamins or minerals may accelerate recovery and/or reduce susceptibility to infections. Some information to confirm these possibilities is available, but confirmatory studies have not been conducted in military populations. As such, if you elect to take supplements, you should monitor your overall health and performance to determine whether the expense is justified. Also, be sure not to take more than 2 to 3 times the RDA; preferably take a supplement that provides nutrients in amounts that meet the RDA (see Chapter 3 for the RDAs).

Vitamin C

> **Supplementation with 600 mg/day of Vitamin C may decrease the incidence of upper respiratory infections during extended missions and/or prolonged activities.**

When selected individuals participate in prolonged competitive athletic events, supplementation with vitamin C has been shown to be beneficial for reducing the incidence and or severity of upper respiratory infections. This may help in BUD/SEAL training, especially during the first phase and Hell Week, when upper respiratory tract infections and cellulitis are frequently noted. Infections, such as an outbreak of pneumococcal pneumonia have also been noted during Ranger training.

Vitamin E

> **Supplementation with 400 IU/day of Vitamin E may protect cell membranes from damage by free radicals produced during strenuous exercise.**

For conditions of altitude exposure, one recent study indicated that mountaineers who took vitamin E supplements minimized altitude-induced performance decrements by being able to maintain adequate blood flow and protect their cell membranes from "oxidative" damage.

Mineral Supplements

As with the vitamins, there is no clear-cut evidence to indicate that mineral supplements will enhance physical performance in normal, healthy individuals. However, some minerals may be useful and others may be harmful.

Chromium

Chromium is becoming increasingly popular among athletes because of purported muscle-building or anabolic effects. The results from studies to date are not consistent, and more work is required before definitive recommendations can be made. Meanwhile, if you take chromium supplements, limit the amount to the current recommendations (200 µg/day); do not take more than 1000 µg/day.

Zinc

Supplementation with zinc has also been studied. Taking a zinc:copper supplement (25 mg to 2 mg) twice a day also seems to minimize the production of free radicals generated during prolonged exercise. However, if zinc supplements are taken, they should provide no more than 100 mg per day, and copper should be taken to prevent a copper deficiency.

Iron

Iron is commonly used by physically active people looking for the performance edge. However, iron supplements do not improve performance in non-deficient individuals. If your diet provides any meat, fish or poultry, it is unlikely you need iron supplements. Moreover, excessive iron intakes can be detrimental (see risks) and **the use of prenatal supplements to boost iron stores is not recommended**.

Antioxidants

As SEALS, you are continually exposed to hazardous environments, extensive sunlight, and other situations which result in a process called "oxidation". Oxidation results in the formation of "Free Radicals" or "Superoxide Anions". Because you are exposed more than the average person, taking an antioxidant supplement may be protective (see chapter 3 for food sources of antioxidants). If you chew tobacco, this may be particularly important to your future health.

Types of Antioxidants

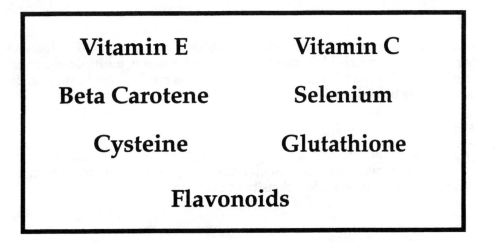

Vitamin E	Vitamin C
Beta Carotene	Selenium
Cysteine	Glutathione
Flavonoids	

◆ Several multivitamin and mineral supplements contain antioxidants - CHECK labels for amounts.

◆ Antioxidant vitamins and minerals are also available as single nutrient supplements, e.g., vitamin E is sold separately. So even if you do not take multivitamins and minerals, you may choose to use an antioxidant.

Risks of Supplementation

The indiscriminate use of high potency vitamins and minerals is of concern since excessive amounts of vitamins and/or minerals can be harmful and may result in nutrient imbalances. Excessive intake of some vitamin and mineral supplements can result in multiple side effects. Harmful side effects of nutrients which are frequently taken in excess are provided on the next page.

Vitamin A

Daily intake of large amounts of vitamin A over several months is extremely toxic. Symptoms of overdosing with retinol include nausea, vomiting, abdominal pain, weight loss, hair loss, cerebral edema (swelling of the brain), and liver failure.

Vitamin B_6

Chronic megadoses of vitamin B_6 have resulted in neurological problems, including loss of muscle coordination and loss of sensation in hands and feet; some individuals may develop these neurological problems with even lower doses of vitamin B_6 (~100 mg/day).

Iron

Chronic use of iron supplements can be a problem, especially in individuals genetically predisposed to iron overload (hemochromatosis); damage to multiple organs including the liver has been observed. Thus, supplemental iron is not indicated unless an iron deficiency anemia has been diagnosed.

Zinc

High intakes of zinc interfere with copper absorption. Daily zinc intakes of >150 mg/day may increase the risk for cardiovascular disease by decreasing serum high density lipoprotein levels and increasing low density lipoprotein levels.

Although some people take excessive amounts of nutrients on a regular basis, it is important to distinguish between excessive and toxic. Intakes of nutrients at their potentially toxic levels can result in significant adverse effects quite readily. Table 4-1 list the toxic values of many nutrients, and these amounts should never be taken. Preferably, intakes will be well below these number, even over a one week period.

Table 4-1. Nutrients and Their Toxicity Values

Nutrient	Toxicity (units/day)	Nutrient	Toxicity (units/day)
Vitamin A	> 25,000 IU	Magnesium	> 6,000 mg
Carotene	None	Boron	>100 mg

Table 4-1. Nutrients and Their Toxicity Values

Nutrient	Toxicity (units/day)	Nutrient	Toxicity (units/day)
Vitamin D	>50,000 IU	Chromium	>10 mg
Vitamin E	>1,200 IU	Copper	>35 mg
Vitamin B$_6$	>2,000 mg	Iron	>100 mg
Vitamin C	Rare	Selenium	>1 mg
Calcium	>2,500 mg	Zinc	>150 mg

What to Look for When Buying Supplements

The better informed you are about marketing practices of vitamin and mineral supplements the more likely you will be to save money and still use a good supplement. For example, did you know that most supplement manufacturers get their initial supply of vitamins and minerals from the same small group of suppliers? After that they formulate their various combinations, label them and sell them. Listed below are some factors you should consider when buying supplements.

Natural Versus Synthetic Vitamins

Both forms are used the same way by the body so why pay more for a "natural" product. Also manufacturers often add a few plant extracts or a bit of the natural vitamin and sell the product at a higher price by labeling it as natural.

Presence of Starch, Sugar, and Other Additives

Many supplements contain starch, binders and other additives. These additives are present in very small amounts and in very rare instances they may cause headaches and other reactions in some people.

Disintegration Rate

If a supplement does not dissolve in the gut, it won't be absorbed and it won't do you any good. One way for you to insure you are taking the right kind of supplement is to look for supplements that meet the U.S. Pharmacopoeia (USP) standards which say that water soluble vitamin supplements should disintegrate in 30 minutes if uncoated and 45 minutes if coated. This standard does not apply to time-release or chewable supplements. Standards for fat-soluble vitamins, minerals and multivitamin are currently being prepared but several companies are already marketing multivitamin-mineral supplements that dissolve within 45 minutes. Look at supplement labels or call the manufacturer for information.

When to Take?

Fat soluble vitamins are better absorbed when taken with food, so if you take a multivitamin/mineral supplement, it is best to take it with a meal.

Tea or coffee will reduce the absorption of several nutrients in supplements.

In general, the body can only absorb and use a certain amounts of nutrients at one time and the rest will be excreted. Do not take a vitamin/mineral supplement with a carbohydrate-protein drink that is already supplemented with vitamins and minerals as you would literally be wasting the supplement and your money.

Amount of Nutrient

Be especially careful about the amount of fat soluble vitamins in the supplement.

Daily supplements should not contain more than 10,000 IU (RDA is 5,000 IU) of Vitamin A as retinol palmitate or acetate.

This form of vitamin A in excess is very toxic. If you use several supplements that each contain retinol palmitate or acetate, you will very quickly exceed safe levels. Also, excessive amounts of the water soluble vitamin, vitamin B_6, can be harmful. Read labels and watch your supplement intakes.

In general, you can safely take 2-3 times the RDA of most vitamins and minerals without harming yourself.

Nutrient Balance

Besides the potential for toxicity, excessive amounts of single nutrient supplements can upset your overall nutrient balance and cause a deficiency in other nutrients. Iron, zinc and copper are good examples since all three are absorbed by the same pathway. An excessive intake of one of these minerals can prevent the proper absorption of the others. This could eventually cause a deficiency and defeat the nutritional enhancement being sought through supplementation.

Expiration Date

The expiration date on labels refers to the length of time a particular supplement is expected to hold its vitamin and mineral potency. Check the expiration date on the label and avoid buying supplements that are due to expire within 6 months since the potency of vitamins may be on the decline.

Summary

◆ Vitamin and/or mineral deficiencies can impair performance. Restoration to a sufficient level reverses performance decrements. However, deficiency states are rare in otherwise healthy males.

◆ Vitamin and mineral supplementation does not improve aerobic capacity, endurance performance, or muscle strength in healthy, nutritionally adequate individuals.

◆ Megadoses of vitamins and /or minerals can be harmful.

◆ CHECK LABELS - to make sure you are not taking too much of any single nutrient.

◆ Under most circumstances you should be able to obtain adequate amounts of vitamins and minerals from your daily diet.

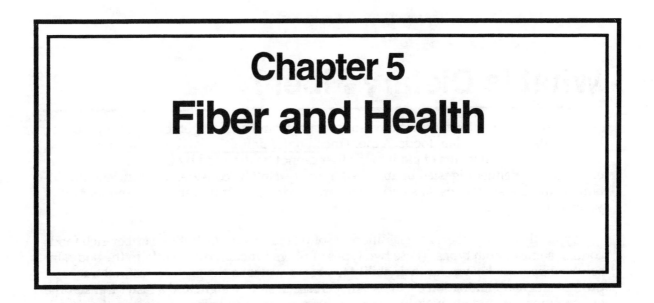

Chapter 5
Fiber and Health

*D*ietary fiber is a food constituent you should be familiar with as it is important for health. Many of the nutritional approaches discussed in this manual will, in fact, promote good health. Although health is important when performance is your end result, you should be aware that dietary fiber should assume a definite BACK SEAT role during mission and training operations/scenarios. In this chapter we will discuss the role of fiber in overall health and during special operations.

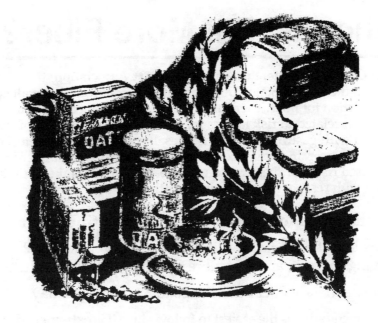

What is Dietary Fiber?

Dietary fiber is a form of carbohydrate we get from fruits, vegetables, grain products, beans, nuts and other plant foods. A more meaningful definition of dietary fiber would be: the structural components of plant foods that cannot be digested by the human body. Because fiber is neither digested or absorbed, it really can't be considered a nutrient, like vitamins, minerals, proteins, fats and other carbohydrates, but it is still an essential part of your diet.

Typically dietary fibers are classified as soluble or insoluble, but most fiber-rich foods contain some of both types. These two types of fibers function differently in the body. Insoluble fibers are known for their ability to absorb water in the gastrointestinal tract and promote regular elimination of stools. An increase in stool weight and a faster transit time are common when diets high in insoluble fiber are ingested. Transit time is the time it takes for your meal to be digested and be excreted in your stools. Insoluble fibers are the predominant fiber in most foods. In contrast, soluble fibers appear to help lower serum cholesterol, a risk factor for heart disease and they also help regulate blood sugar levels. These special effects of dietary fiber have prompted many health promotion agencies to make specific recommendations regarding how much dietary fiber our diet should provide. In a nutshell, fiber serves a very important role in health.

Why Should I Eat More Fiber?

The National Cancer Institute, the American Heart Association, the National Academy of Sciences, and the United States Department of Agriculture have all come out with dietary recommendation for fiber. There are many reasons to increase your daily intake of fiber, and they are all related to risk factors for chronic disease. A lack of fiber in the diet has been associated with gastrointestinal diseases, hypertension, diabetes, heart disease, and several types of cancer, including colon cancer, whereas a high fiber intake is associated with a decreased risk. For these reasons, increasing your intake of dietary fiber may be very important with respect to your future health.

Recommendations for intake of dietary fiber include:

◆ Consume at least 3 - 5 servings of various vegetables, 2 or more servings of fruit, and 6 or more servings of grain products, or

◆ Increase dietary fiber intake to 20 to 35 grams per day

The first recommendation is the easiest to follow since it is extremely difficult to know how much fiber is in each food. Moreover, what the above mentioned organizations use as a typical serving is probably only a quarter of what your portions are. For example, one serving of fruit would be one apple, one banana, one orange or one pear. One serving of grain products would be one slice of whole wheat bread or one bagel. Furthermore, one serving of vegetables would be 1/2 cup of peas, one small potato, or 1/2 cup of carrots. It is likely that you are eating more than one serving at each meal.

How Can I Get More Fiber in My Diet?

Eating more fruits and vegetables, whole wheat breads, whole grain cereals, beans, rice, nuts and seeds is the best way to add fiber to your diet. Foods that provide the most soluble fiber include kidney beans, avocados, green beans, baked potatoes with their skin, sweet potatoes, oatmeal, oranges, bananas, and watermelon. A list of some foods and their total dietary fiber in grams (g) is provided below.

Table 5-1. Serving Sizes and Dietary Fiber Content (in grams) of Selected Foods

Fruits			Vegetables		
Apple	1 medium	2.0	Asparagus, cooked	4 spears	1.5
Banana	1 medium	1.5	Green Beans, cooked	1 cup	2.4
Cantaloupe	1/2 medium	1.9	Broccoli, cooked	1 cup	5.4
Grapefruit	1/2 medium	0.6	Brussels Sprouts, cooked	1 cup	6.4
Grapes	20 each	1.0	Carrots, raw	1 medium	1.8
Orange	1 medium	2.5	Corn, cooked	1 ear	1.6
Pear, Bartlett	1 medium	4.6	Green Pepper, raw	1 whole	1.3
Plum	1 each	0.8	Potato, baked with skin	1 medium	5.1
Raisins	1/2 cup	2.6	Potato, french fries	20 fries	4.6
Watermelon	1 cup	0.6	Sweet Potato, baked with skin	1 medium	3.4

Table 5-1. Serving Sizes and Dietary Fiber Content (in grams) of Selected Foods

Breads, Cereals and Grain Products			Legumes, Nuts, Seeds, and Miscellaneous		
Bread, French	2 slices	1.9	Almonds	2 tbsp	2.5
Bread, Whole Wheat	2 slices	1.3	Avocado	1/2 medium	4.7
English Muffin	1 whole	0.9	Black-eyed peas, cooked	1 cup	7.1
Saltine Cracker	10 squares	1.7	Green Peas, cooked	1 cup	6.0
Taco Shell	2 each	4.4	Kidney Beans, cooked	1 cup	5.8
Corn Flakes	1 cup	1.0	Lima Beans, cooked	1 cup	7.1
All Bran	1 cup	9.1	Peanut Butter	2 tbsp	2.0
Shredded Wheat	1 cup	5.5	Walnuts	2 tbsp	1.1
Rice, cooked	1 cup	0.7			
Spaghetti, cooked	1 cup	1.9			

When Should I Minimize My Fiber Intake?

Dietary fiber is very important to your health: it promotes regularity by increasing stool bulk and weight. However, during extended operations, you will most likely want to avoid "regular eliminations" for as long as possible. A low fiber diet may be preferred for these occasions. Also, many high fiber foods can cause bloating and gas if you are not accustomed to eating them or if you don't drink enough water. Make sure to try such foods during training so you can find out how your system reacts. That way you can make dietary modifications where necessary before the actual event.

For Special Operations You May Want to Minimize Your Intake of Dietary Fiber

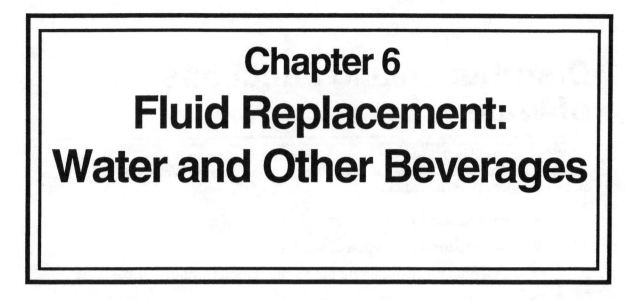

Chapter 6
Fluid Replacement:
Water and Other Beverages

Water is an essential nutrient and the most abundant component of the human body. Believe it or not, approximately 60% of your total body weight is water. Since lean body/muscle mass requires more water than fat, the leaner you are, the more body water you have. As you may imagine, water must be consumed regularly to ensure normal functioning of your body.

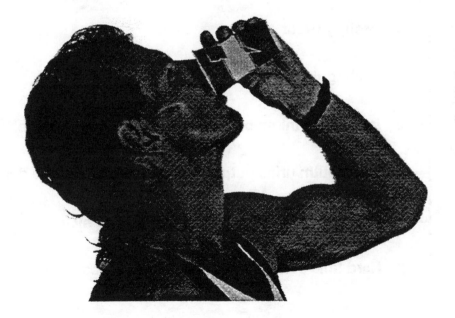

Distribution and Functions of Water

Water is found both inside and outside cells, but most water is inside cells, especially muscle cells. The lowest concentration of water is in bone and fat. Water in the body serves many important roles, including:

◆   Participates in digestion and absorption of nutrients

◆   Participates in excretion of wastes

◆   Essential for maintaining blood circulation throughout the body

◆   Maintains body temperature

A loss of 20% of body water can result in death, and if 4% of your body weight is lost because of sweating, large decrements in decision-making, concentration, and physical work occur. In addition, being well hydrated during operations is absolutely critical, since adequate fluid volume will help compensate for blood loss when wounded. For these reasons, consumption of water is absolutely critical, and maintenance of water balance is essential to SEAL performance. Below are signs and symptoms you might experience as you become dehydrated.

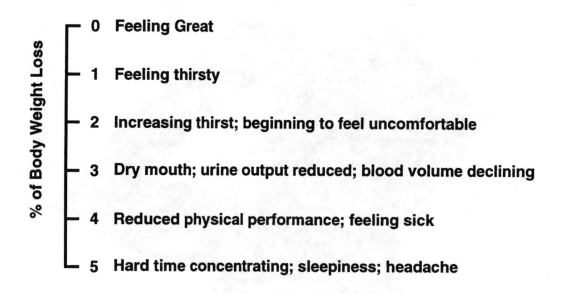

% of Body Weight Loss

0   **Feeling Great**

1   **Feeling thirsty**

2   **Increasing thirst; beginning to feel uncomfortable**

3   **Dry mouth; urine output reduced; blood volume declining**

4   **Reduced physical performance; feeling sick**

5   **Hard time concentrating; sleepiness; headache**

How to Maintain Water Balance

Water balance is determined by water/fluid output and input. In order to maintain performance, it is critical that a fluid deficit, or dehydration does not occur. With dehydration, water output exceeds input and balance becomes negative. The average man loses 1,000 ml to 2,300 ml (0.9 to 2.4 quarts) of water/day. This water is lost:

◆ In the urine

◆ Through breathing

◆ By sweating

◆ Through the stools.

When activity level is low, most fluids are lost through the urine. However, when activity level or the outdoor temperature is high, most fluid is lost by sweating. In fact, up to 2,000 ml (1.8 quarts) per hour can be lost through sweating, depending on outside temperatures.

All fluids lost must be added back to the body each day to maintain fluid balance. Sources of fluid for the body are:

◆ Water in food

◆ Water in beverages (like orange juice, coffee, sodas and beer)

◆ Water from the metabolism or chemical breakdown of foods

The easiest way to restore fluid balance is by drinking water, and this is *VERY* important to remember. The figure on the next page graphically depicts water output and input for normal temperature conditions, hot weather, and with prolonged exercise. Notice how sweat output increases dramatically with both hot weather and prolonged exercise - these amounts would be even greater if exercise were performed in the heat. The only way to match this great output is to drink fluids.

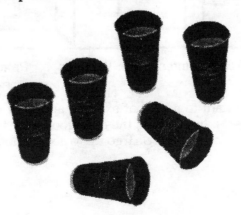

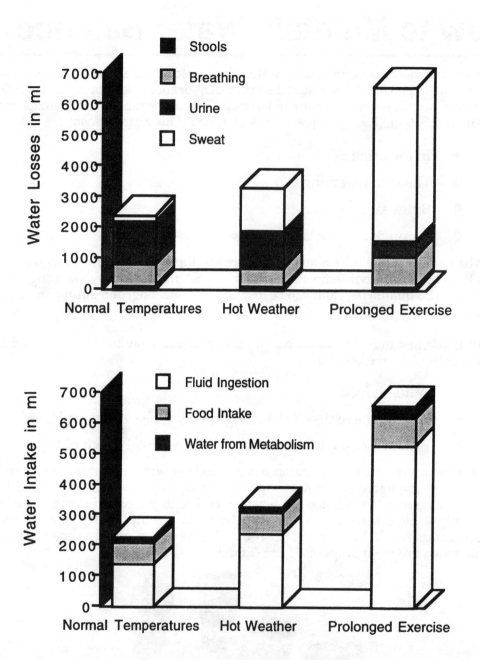

In this figure it is important to note that exercise and heat exposure increase sweat losses and reduce urine losses. In addition, the only good way to replace those "lost fluids" is by drinking fluids: fluid intake MUST go up to accommodate losses.

Although eating fods high in water will help restore or maintain water balance, drinking fluids is preferred. Some foods that are over 90% water, include watermelon, strawberries, grapefruit, cucumbers, and many other fresh fruits and vegetables. If you eat many of those foods and drink lots of beverages, it is less likely you would be in negative water balance.

What Conditions Will Increase Water Losses?

The primary factors which could cause dehydration are:

◆ Exercising for over 30 minutes

◆ Working in a hot environment - wet or dry

◆ Working in a cold environment - wet or dry

◆ Going to high altitudes

◆ Drinking too much alcohol

◆ Exercising in the heat, cold, or at altitude

◆ Exercising with a hangover

How Can You Make Sure to Get Enough Fluids?

Several points about fluid intake should be considered:

◆ Do not rely on thirst as a good indicator of fluid needs; body weight losses are better

◆ Before any exercise or simulated-mission, you should drink fluids, in anticipation of losing fluid

◆ Before you start, make sure your urine is clear (unless you take B vitamin supplements) - this is a sign that you are well hydrated. The more dehydrated you are, the darker (and smellier) your urine will be

- Drink regularly or whenever possible during your workouts and operations

- Weigh yourself before and after an event to determine how much fluid you have lost - for every pound of weight lost, you should drink 16 ounces of fluid (2 cups or 500 ml)

What You Should Drink

Many beverages - both regular and sports drinks - are commercially available. These include:

Carbohydrate/Electrolyte Drinks	**Fruit Juices**
Carbonated Beverages	**Water**

Although the type of activity you participate in will determine what you drink, the beverage you select should:

- Taste good

- Cause no gastrointestinal/stomach discomfort

- Be rapidly absorbed

- Contain sodium and potassium especially when exercising for a prolonged period in the heat

- Have an osmolality of less than 350 mOsm/L

Osmolality refers to the number of particles in solution. If it is high (> 350), the beverage can cause stomach distress and not be absorbed well if you drink it shortly before or during physical activity. Note in the chart below that the osmolality of some beverages is greater than 350. Thus, if you choose to drink those beverages as sports drinks, you should dilute them appropriately or drink an equal amount of water. For example, orange juice should be mixed with an equal amount of water.

If the exercise is of long duration, it may be advisable to ingest a beverage that provides energy in the form of carbohydrate (CHO) to the working muscles. Beverages with "glucose polymers", which are complex CHOs are usually preferred over the glucose and sucrose drinks, which are simple CHOs. However, the important message is to drink. Below is a list of beverages, some of which are currently used as "fluid replacement beverages" by athletes and others that are popular with many individuals.

Table 6-1. Comparison of Fluid Replacement Beverages

Beverage*	CHO Source[1] & Concentration	Sodium (mg)	Potassium (mg)	Other Nutrients	Osmolality (mOsm/L)
Gatorade®	6% Sucrose/Glucose	110	25	Chloride, Phosphorus	280-360
Exceed®	7.2% Glucose Polymers/Fructose	50	45	Chloride, Calcium, Magnesium, Phosphorus	250
Body Fuel®	4.2% Maltodextrin/ Fructose	80	20	Phosphorous, Chloride, Iron, Vitamins A, B, & C	210
10-K®	6.3% Sucrose/Glucose/ Fructose	52	26	Phosphorous, Vitamin C, Chloride	350
Quickick®	4.7% Fructose/Sucrose	116	23	Calcium, Chloride, Phosphorous	305
Coca Cola	11% High Fructose Corn Syrup/Sucrose	9.2	trace	Phosphorus	600-715
Sprite	10.2% High Fructose Corn Syrup/Sucrose	28	trace	----	695
Cranberry Juice Cocktail	15% High Fructose Corn Syrup/Sucrose	10	61	Vitamin C, Phosphorus	890
Orange Juice	11.8% Fructose/ Sucrose/Glucose	2.7	510	Calcium, Niacin, Iron, Vitamins A & C, Thiamin, Phosphorus, Riboflavin	690
Water	-----	low	low	low	10-20

*Serving Size = 8 fluid ounces.

[1]Sucrose = fructose and glucose; Maltodextrin = a mixture of short chains (2 - 3 molecules linked) of glucose; high fructose corn syrup = a 54:46% mixture of fructose and glucose derived from processed and converted corn starch; glucose polymers = long chains (> 3 molecules linked) of glucose.

When and How Much to Drink?

Remember: the following recommendations are generally sound for most people. However, everyone is different so you must learn to look for signs alerting you to **your** fluid needs. Also, you need to make adjustments depending on the temperature outside. If it is very hot, you may need to double the recommendations. Remember the more active you are the more fluid you need. Be careful not to drink TOO much plain water, especially during prolonged exercise in the heat.

Table 6-2. Fluid Intake Recommendations for Before, During and After an Event or Mission

	TYPE OF FLUID	FREQUENCY	VOLUME
High intensity activities shorter than 1 hour (soccer game, PT test, 10k run)			
BEFORE[1]	5-8% Beverage with CHO[2]	1 - 2 hours before	8 - 16 oz. (1 - 2 cups)
DURING	Water	As needed	16 - 32 oz. (2 - 4 cups)
AFTER	5-8% Beverage with CHO[1]	0 to 2 hours after	16 - 32 oz. - Check your weight since you may need more
Moderate to high intensity activities lasting 1 to 3 hours (long run, swim, or march)			
BEFORE[1]	Water	0 to 2 hours before	8 - 16 oz. per hour
DURING	5-8% Beverage with CHO and electrolytes	Every 20 to 30 minutes	12 - 24 oz. per 30 minutes
AFTER	5-8% Beverage with CHO and electrolytes	0 - 2 hours after	8 - 16 oz. per 30 minutes - Check your weight since you may need more

Table 6-2. Fluid Intake Recommendations for Before, During and After an Event or Mission

	TYPE OF FLUID	FREQUENCY	VOLUME
Low to moderate intensity activities lasting over 3 hours (land warfare scenario)			
BEFORE[1]	Water	0 - 2 hours before	8 - 16 oz. per hour
DURING	5 - 8% Beverage with CHO and electrolytes	Every 20 to 30 minutes	8 - 16 oz. per 30 minutes
AFTER	5 - 8% Beverage with CHO and electrolytes	0 - 6 hours after	8 - 16 oz. every 30 minutes - Check your weight since you may need more
Low to moderate intensity activities in the water for less than 3 hours (short dives)			
BEFORE[1]	Water	0 - 1 hour before	12 - 16 oz.
DURING - If possible	Water or a 5 - 8% Beverage with CHO	Every hour	8 - 16 oz. per hour
AFTER	5 - 8% Beverage with CHO	0 - 2 hours after	16 - 32 oz. per hour - Check your weight since you may need more

Table 6-2. Fluid Intake Recommendations for Before, During and After an Event or Mission

	TYPE OF FLUID	FREQUENCY	VOLUME
Low intensity activities in the water for more than 3 hours (long dives or SDV operation)			
BEFORE[1]	Water	0 - 1 hour before	12 - 16 oz.
DURING - If possible	5 - 8% Beverage with CHO	Every hour	16 oz. per hour
AFTER	5 - 8% Beverage with CHO	0 - 6 hours after	16 - 32 oz.per hour - Check your weight since you may need more

[1] In all cases, you should have had sufficient fluid to produce a clear, pale urine (unless you are taking vitamin B supplements), and you should weigh yourself before and after to monitor fluid losses.

[2] CHO stands for carbohydrate such as found in the beverages already described.

Table 6-3. Typical Fluid Losses for Various Events

Event	Duration of Event (hrs)	Typical Fluid Losses (qts)
Typical Day at BUDs	12	10
Working in the Heat	8	6.3
Diving in Cold Water	6	1.4
Working in MOPP Gear	4	6.4
SDV Operation	3-7	2.1
5.5 Mile Swim Wearing Full Body Wet Suit	4	3.2

Table 6-3. Typical Fluid Losses for Various Events

Event	Duration of Event (hrs)	Typical Fluid Losses (qts)
2-Day Hike In Cold Weather	3	2.6
Triathalon	4	3.2
Marathon	3.5	3.7

Table 6-4. Determining Amounts of Fluid and CHO to Drink During Exercise

The approximate number of 8 ounce cups of fluid required to provide varying amounts of carbohydrate (CHO) each hour for a given concentration of CHO in the beverage is presented below. Beverage concentrations are on the left (3% to 12%) and the amount of CHO delivered per hour is across the top (20 to 60 gm). For example, if you want to consume 40 grams of CHO each hour and the weather is hot, you may wish to make up a 5% rather than an 8% solution so you are drinking 3.5 cups instead of 2 cups of fluid. This is important because you need more fluid in the heat.

Concentration of Beverage	Carbohydrate Delivered by Beverage of Given Concentration				
	20 gm/hr	30 gm/hr	40 gm/hr	50 gm/hr	60 gm/hr
	Approximate Volumes (cups) of Beverage Required to Deliver CHO/hr[1]				
3%	3	4	6	7	8.5
5%	2	2.5	3.5	4	5
7%	1	2	2.5	3	3.5
8%	1	1.5	2	2.5	3
10%	1	1.25	2	2	2.5
12%	1	1	1.5	2	2

[1] The shaded section represents the volumes of beverage that are adequate for fluid replacement (2 to 5 cups/hr). The unshaded sections are volumes that are either too low (< 2 cups/hr) or too high (>5 cups/hr) to confer any benefit.

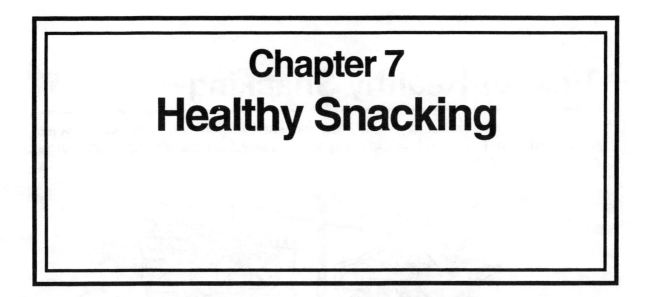

Chapter 7
Healthy Snacking

*S*nacking, "eating between regular meals", can be extremely important when it comes to performing your duties and assignments. Your energy expenditure can be extremely high on given days and during various operations, and it is often difficult to eat enough at meals. Snacking becomes very important during this time. In addition, you probably snack at various times during the day and evening anyway, so it becomes important to look at what constitutes healthy snacks. Most people think snacking is unhealthy and leads to weight gain, but that notion has emerged because most people don't eat healthy snacks! If you don't care about gaining weight, just about any snack will do, but if you want to maintain weight and perform well, then selection of snacks is critical.

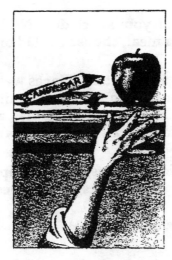

Tips for Healthy Snacking

Think through a typical day. How often and where do you usually snack? Are your snacks healthy or loaded with fat? In case you aren't sure, here are some tips to help promote health snacking!

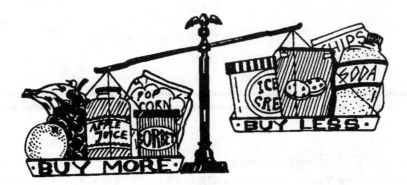

Stock your cupboards and refrigerator with plain popcorn, whole grain crackers, Dutch pretzels, unsweetened fruit juices, fresh fruits and vegetables, and lowfat yogurt and cheeses.

Carry naturally sweet fresh fruits, such as grapes, a pear, apple, or watermelon, for a snack rather than candy or cookies.

Limit the amount eaten so your snack does NOT replace a meal. If it is taking the place of a meal, choose a salad or healthy sandwich.

Choose a snack that provides dietary fiber as well as other nutrients (unless the snack is for a mission). Fresh fruits with edible seeds (berries) or skins (apples, peaches, plums, pears), raw vegetables, and whole grain pretzels or crackers are all good sources of fiber.

Try eating dried apricots, bananas, apples, figs, dates, pineapples, and prunes.

Make a snack mix with wheat, rice, and corn ready-to-eat cereals.

Eat raw vegetables such as celery with lowfat cheese spreads.

Table 7-1. Macronutrient Composition of Selected Snacks

FOOD	Serving Size	Approximate amount per Serving				
		Energy (Kcal)	CHO (grams)	Protein (grams)	Fat (grams)	Fiber (grams)
Breads, Cereals, and Other Grain Products						
Angel Food Cake	1 piece	129	29.3	3.0	0.1	ND[1]
Bagel	1 each	200	38.0	7.5	1.1	1.5
Cornnuts®	2 oz.	249	41.6	4.8	8.0	6.9
Crackers, whole wheat	8-2" squares	70	10.0	1.6	4.0	1
Crackers, Saltines	4 squares	50	8.0	1.0	1.0	0.3
Crackers, Round Snack	4 each	60	7.0	1.0	4.0	0.2
English Muffin with Raisins	1 whole	137	27.5	4.3	1.5	0.9
Fig Newtons	2 cookies	112	23.0	1.2	2.4	1.5
Graham Crackers	2 squares	60	11.0	1.0	1.4	0.4
Granola Bars, plain	1 bar	115	15.8	2.5	4.9	ND
Muffins, Blueberry	2.5" dia	158	27.0	3.2	4.0	2.1
Muffin, Bran	2.5" dia	154	27.5	4.0	6.0	4.3
Popcorn, plain - air popped	1 cup	30	6.2	1.0	trace	1.2
Popcorn, buttered	1 cup	55	6.3	1.0	3.1	1.1
Pretzels Dutch, hard, plain	2 each	130	26.0	4.0	1.0	ND
Pretzel Sticks, thin, salted	10 each	210	48.0	6.0	2.0	ND

Table 7-1. Macronutrient Composition of Selected Snacks

FOOD	Serving Size	Approximate amount per Serving				
		Energy (Kcal)	CHO (grams)	Protein (grams)	Fat (grams)	Fiber (grams)
Sports Bars						
Pure Power	2.3 oz.	240	42.0	12.0	3.0	2.0
Pro-Sports	2.3 oz.	140	40.0	15.0	2.0	ND
Tiger Sport	2.3 oz.	230	40.0	11.0	3.0	ND
Twin Labs Amino Fuel	2.7 oz.	285	50.0	15.0	3.0	ND
Clif by Avocet	2.4 oz.	250	53.0	6.0	3.0	8.0
Cross Trainer	2.25 oz.	236	46.0	11.0	2.0	ND
Exceed Bar	2.9 oz.	280	53.0	12.0	2.0	3.0
Meal on the GO	3 oz.	290	51.0	7.0	9.0	ND
Power Bar	2.25 oz.	225	40.0	10.0	2.0	2.0
Vegetables						
Carrot Sticks	1 large	30	7.0	1.0	0.0	1.8
Cauliflower	1 cup	25	5.0	2.0	0.0	2.3
Cucumbers	6 slices	5	1.0	trace	0.0	0.2
Potatoes, French Fries	10 fries	110	17.0	2.0	4.0	1.2
Tomato Juice	1 cup	40	10.0	2.0	0.0	ND

Table 7-1. Macronutrient Composition of Selected Snacks

FOOD	Serving Size	Approximate amount per Serving				
		Energy (Kcal)	CHO (grams)	Protein (grams)	Fat (grams)	Fiber (grams)
Fruits						
Apple	1 medium	80	21.0	trace	trace	2.8
Apricot, Dried	7 halves	80	20.0	1.0	0.0	ND
Banana	1 medium	105	22.0	0.0	1.0	22.0
Cantaloupe	1 half	95	22.0	2.0	0.5	1.8
Orange	1 medium	60	15.0	1.0	trace	2.4
Raisins	1/2 cup	218	57.0	2.5	0.5	2.6
Fruit Cocktail in Juice Pack	1 cup	115	29.0	1.0	trace	ND
Fruit Leather	1 bar	81	18.0	0.4	1.2	ND
Watermelon	1 cup	50	11.0	1.0	trace	0.6
Sweets And Other Snacks						
Beef Jerky	1 large piece	280	2.9	7.9	2.6	ND
Fruit Shake (see recipe at end)	1 serving	330	60	15.0	3.0	ND
Fruit Yogurt, lowfat	1 cup, 8 oz.	230	43	10.0	2.0	ND
Popsicles	1 - 3 oz.	70	18	0.0	0.0	ND

[1]ND = No Data

What Snacks are Best for Different Occasions?

In the following charts, examples of snacks are provided. Some of the snacks are part of military rations, and should (could) be used during training or mission maneuvers. Other snacks may not be realistic in the field, but are good choices if you are able to be more selective in what you choose.

Operations at Night

If you need to stay up at night you should select a snack that is *low in fat, high in carbohydrate (CHO), and provides some or a moderate amount of protein.* You want to avoid foods that are 100% CHO. Sports bars would be ideal snacks for night operations. Also, crackers (or other forms of bread) with egg salad, mashed beans, jelly, tuna, or low fat cream cheese, would be suitable. Finally, some of the protein/CHO beverages described in Chapter 6 would be suitable for night time operations.

Table 7-2. Snacks to Eat During Night Time Operations

Sports Bars	**Fruit Bars**
Oatmeal Cookie Bars	**Protein/CHO Beverage**
Trail Mix	**Crackers with Jelly or Cheese**

Exercises in the Heat

The ideal snacks consumed during strenuous activities in warm to hot environments are those which provide the body with fluid. As such, fruits, especially watermelon and oranges are great snack for hot weather. Otherwise, the fluid replacement beverages described in Chapter 6 are preferred. Avoid high fat and dried foods which can make you uncomfortable and thirsty.

Table 7-3. Snacks to Eat During Exercises in the Heat

Watermelon	Oranges
Applesauce	Fruit Popsicles
Grapes	CHO Beverages with Electrolytes

Exercises in the Cold

When working in cold weather, snack on foods that are high in CHO. CHO foods produce more heat when digested than either fat or protein. To go along with your food snack, a hot beverage, like cocoa or soup, would be great.

Table 7-4. Snacks to Eat During Exercises in the Cold

Granola/Sport Bars	Fig Newtons
Hot Chocolate	Crackers/Bread with Jam
Fruit Bars	Chicken Noodle Soup
Trail Mix	Hot Apple Cider

Sustained Operations

By definition, SUSTAINED OPERATIONS are those missions or training sessions where you must work continuously for over 24 hours with minimal sleep, and few rest periods. During these times it is important to receive adequate amounts of CHO to maintain your "blood glucose" and fluid to maintain "hydration status". The specific types of snacks will depend on the temperature and how long you have been working, but in general avoid high fat foods since they take longer to digest than CHO foods. Also, eating CHO with some protein will help you stay awake when you are feeling drowsy. A combination of the recommendations already made in this chapter would be best, depending on the environmental conditions.

Table 7-5. Snacks to Eat During Sustained Operations

Granola/Power Bars	Oatmeal Cookies
Hot or Cold Protein/ CHO Beverage	Cracker/Bread with Jam
M & M's	Trail Mix
Tootsie Roll	Dried Fruit

Snacking On Occasion

There comes a time when you just don't want to be healthy - you want to get some quick energy and nothing else. In that case it is still wise to be selective, so if you must have a candy bar or other sweets, choose one that is high in CHO and as low in fat as possible: like Peppermint Patties and 3 Musketeers. Remember, these foods are not encouraged because they provide ONLY energy - no vitamins or minerals, which you must have to process the energy. BUT sweets now and then will certainly NOT hurt you.

Table 7-6. Macronutrient Composition of Some Sweet Snacks

Candy Bars and Sweet Items	ENERGY (kcal)	CHO (grams)	FAT (% of Energy)	CHO (% of Energy)
Almond Joy, 1.76 oz. bar	232	29	51	45
Baby Ruth, 2.1 oz. bar	277	37	40	52
Butterfinger Bar, 2.16 oz. bar	266	41	36	58
Chocolate Coated Raisins, 1.58 oz. pkg	188	32	33	61
Gumdrops, 10 small	135	35	0	100
Jelly Beans, 10 small	40	10	0	100
Kit Kat, 1.625 oz. bar	235	28	49	46
Milky Way Bar, 2.1 oz. bar	251	43	32	64
3 Musketeers, 2.13 oz. bar	249	46	27	70
M & M's Plain, 1.69 oz. pkg	229	33	40	54
M & M's Peanut, 1.74 oz. pkg	242	29	47	45
Peppermint Pattie, 1 large	149	34	22	74
Snickers, 2.16 oz. bar	277	37	42	51
Tootsie Roll, 1 oz.	112	23	19	78

Snack Recipes

Fruit Shake

1 cup ice cubes
1 cup skim milk
1 ripe banana
2 Peaches or 1/2 to 1 cup of any fresh fruit
2 Tbsp almonds
1 Tbsp honey
2 tsp wheat germ

Place all ingredients in a blender or food processor and blend until smooth. For extra protein add 1/4 cup of non-fat dried milk. Makes 1 serving.

Nutrition Information: 520 kcal, 70% CHO, 12% Protein, and 18% Fat per serving.

Trail Mix

3 cup seedless raisins
1 cup dried apricots
1 cup dried apples
1 cup almonds
1 cup dry roasted peanuts
1 cup dried pineapple
1 cup dried dates
1/2 cup sunflower seeds

Mix all ingredients together in large bowl or bag. Makes 10 -1 cup servings.
Nutrition Information: 560 kcal, 62% CHO, 7% Protein, and 30% Fat per 1 cup serving.

Chapter 8
Restaurants, Fast Foods and Eating Out

*T*he average American eats one of three meals away from home each day, and it is likely that many of you are eating 5, 6, 7 or more meals a week away from home. Learning how to "eat out" is very important if you want to optimize your performance. You are probably aware that eating out presents different problems than eating at home. When we talk about eating out we mean eating at restaurants, fast food places, on travel, on vacations, and at social events.

Most people love to eat in restaurants or at places away from home. Eating out provides a change in routine, an opportunity to try new foods, a chance to socialize and a break from cooking and washing dishes (for those who do). Restaurant and fast food meals do not have to be unhealthy. By being informed and by asking appropriate questions, you can stay within the guidelines of your nutrition program and still enjoy the benefits of eating out.

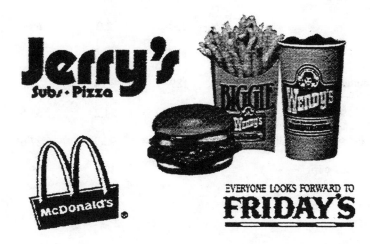

Fast Food Restaurants

Although we don't encourage you to get your meals from fast food establishments, we know fast foods are a way of life. If you could learn to select the types of foods that will suit your activity patterns and performance requirements, then fast food restaurants are OK. Below are selected foods typically available at different fast food places, and the energy, carbohydrate (CHO), and fat contributions of those foods. After providing you with this information, sample breakfasts and lunch/dinners that maybe considered nutritionally adequate in terms of their CHO and fat content are presented.

Table 8-1. Caloric Values of Selected Fast Foods

Breakfast Items	Energy (kcal)	CHO (grams)	Fat (% of Energy)	CHO (% of Energy)
Hot Chocolate, 6 oz.	103	22.5	9.6	87.4
Orange Juice, 8 oz.	112	26.8	0.0	95.7
Biscuit, 1 plain	276	34.4	43.7	49.9
Biscuit w/ egg	315	24.2	57.7	30.7
Biscuit w/ egg and sausage	582	41.2	59.8	28.3
Croissant w/ egg and cheese	369	24.3	60.2	26.3
Cinnamon Danish, 1 medium	349	46.9	43.1	53.8
Eggs, 2 scrambled	200	2.0	68.4	4.0
English Muffin, 1 plain	137	27.5	6.6	80.3
English Muffin w/ butter	189	36.4	27.6	77.0
English Muffin w/ cheese and sausage	394	24.2	55.5	24.6
Pancakes w/ butter and syrup, 3 medium	519	90.9	27.6	77.0
Potatoes, hashed brown, 1 cup	302	32.3	55.5	24.6

Table 8-1. Caloric Values of Selected Fast Foods

Lunch and Dinner Items	Energy (kcal)	CHO (grams)	Fat (% of Energy)	CHO (% of Energy)
Chocolate Shake 10 oz.	360	57.9	26.3	64.3
Cola 12 oz.	151	37.6	0.0	99.6
Burrito w/ Bean, 2 each	448	71.4	27.1	63.8
Burrito w/ Beef, 2 each	523	58.5	35.8	44.7
Chili Con Carne, 1 cup	254	21.9	29.4	34.5
Cheeseburger, double meat, 1 each	416	35.2	45.6	33.8
Fish Sandwich, 1 each	524	47.6	49.1	36.3
Chicken, breast fried, 2 pieces	494	35.7	65.0	15.4
Hot Dog w/ chili, 1 each	297	31.3	40.6	42.2
Nachos w/ cheese, 7 each	345	36.3	51.1	42.1
Pizza w/ cheese, 2 slices	218	31.9	20.6	58.5
Taco, 1 large	569	41.1	50.0	28.9
Onion Rings, 10 each	332	37.7	50.7	45.4
Potato Chips, 10 each	105	10.4	60.9	39.6
Potatoes, French Fries, 1 order	237	29.3	46.3	49.5
Salad w/out dressing, 1 1/2 cups	32	6.7	0.0	83.8
Potato, baked w/sour cream, 1 medium	394	50.0	49.8	44.4
Corn w/butter, 1 ear	155	32	9.7	82.6
Coleslaw, 3/4 cup	147	12.8	67.3	34.8
Brownies, 1 each	243	39.o	37.4	64.2
Chocolate Chip Cookies, 1 order	233	36.2	42.1	52.8
Hot Fudge Sundae	284	47.7	31.2	78.6
Fried Fruit Pie, 1 each	266	33.1	48.7	49.8

Table 8-2. Sample High Carbohydrate Fast Food Breakfasts, Lunches and Dinners

MacDonald's Breakfast	Energy (kcal)	CHO (grams)	Fat (% of Energy)	CHO (% of Energy)
Orange Juice, 8 oz.	112	26.8	0.0	93.8
2 English Muffins w/jam or honey	378	72.8	27.6	77.0
Eggs, 2 scrambled	200	2.0	68.4	4.0
Hot Chocolate	103	22.5	9.6	87.4
Total	**793**	**124.1**	**31.7**	**62.6**

Wendy's Breakfast

	Energy (kcal)	CHO (grams)	Fat (% of Energy)	CHO (% of Energy)
Orange Juice, 16 oz.	224	53.6	0.0	93.8
Cinnamon Danish, 2 medium	698	93.8	43.1	53.8
Hot Chocolate, 6oz.	100	22.0	9.0	88.0
Total	**1022**	**169.4**	**30.3**	**66.3**

Anywhere Breakfast 1

	Energy (kcal)	CHO (grams)	Fat (% of Energy)	CHO (% of Energy)
Orange Juice, 8 oz.	112	26.8	0.0	93.8
Pancakes w/ butter and syrup 3 medium	692	121.2	25.3	70.1
Eggs, 2 scrambled	200	2.0	68.4	4.0
Hot Chocolate, 6 oz.	103	22.5	9.6	87.4
Total	**1107**	**172.2**	**29.0**	**62.2**

Burger King Breakfast	Energy (kcal)	CHO (grams)	Fat (% of Energy)	CHO (% of Energy)
Orange Juice, 16 oz.	224	53.6	0.0	93.8
Egg Croissantwich, 1 each	369	24.3	60.2	26.3
Hot chocolate, 6 oz	100	22.0	9.0	88.0
Total	**693**	**99.3**	**33.3**	**57.7**

Anywhere Breakfast 2

	Energy (kcal)	CHO (grams)	Fat (% of Energy)	CHO (% of Energy)
Orange Juice, 16 oz.	224	53.6	0.0	93.8
English Muffin, 2 with 2 pkg jam	342	73.0	5.2	85.3
Eggs, 2 scrambled	200	2.0	68.4	4.0
Hash Brown Potatoes, 1 cup	302	32.3	53.6	42.8
Total	**1068**	**161.0**	**30.0**	**60.3**

Taco Bell Lunch or Dinner

	Energy (kcal)	CHO (grams)	Fat (% of Energy)	CHO (% of Energy)
Taco Bell Nachos, 2 orders	692	75.0	48.1	43.4
Cola, 16 oz	201	50.1	0.0	99.8
Total	**893**	**125.1**	**36.7**	**56.0**

Anywhere Lunch or Dinner	Energy (kcal)	CHO (grams)	Fat (% of Energy)	CHO (% of Energy)
Chili Con Carne, 1 cup	254	21.9	29.4	34.5
Potato, baked, plain, 1 medium	300	69.0	0.5	92.0
Sour Cream, 1pkt	60	1.0	90.0	6.7
Green Salad , tossed, 1 1/2 cups	32	6.7	0.0	83.8
Italian Dressing, reduced calorie, 2 Tbsp	50	3.0	72.0	24.0
Corn on cob, 2 ears	310	64.0	19.7	82.6
Chocolate Shake, 10 oz.	360	57.9	26.3	64.3
Total	**1366**	**223.5**	**24.8**	**65.4**

Wendy's Lunch or Dinner

	Energy (kcal)	CHO (grams)	Fat (% of Energy)	CHO (% of Energy)
Fettucine, 2 cups	480	60	29.7	48.8
Spaghetti Sauce, 1 cup	120	24	0	77.4
Garlic Toast, 1 serving	140	18	38.6	51.4
Caesar Salad, 1 serving	160	18	45.0	45.0
Lemonade, 16 oz.	200	50	0	100
Total	**1100**	**170**	**24.5**	**61.8**

Hardee's Lunch or Dinner

	Energy (kcal)	CHO (grams)	Fat (% of Energy)	CHO (% of Energy)
Big Roast Beef Sandwich, 1 serving	346	33.5	35.8	38.7
Potato, baked, plain, 1 medium	300	69.0	0.5	92
Sour Cream, 1pkt	60	1.0	90.0	6.7
Green Salad, tossed, 1 1/2 cups	32	6.7	0.0	83.8
French Dressing, low fat, 2 Tbsp	44	7.0	36.0	63.6
Vanilla Shake, 10 oz.	314	50.8	24.1	64.7
Total	**1096**	**168.0**	**24.7**	**61.3**

Pizza Hut Lunch or Dinner	Energy (kcal)	CHO (grams)	Fat (% of Energy)	CHO (% of Energy)
Pizza w/ cheese, 8 slices	872	127.6	20.6	58.5
Salad w/out dressing, 1 1/2 cups	32	6.7	0.0	83.8
Italian Dressing, reduced calorie, 2 Tbsp	50	3.0	72.0	24.0
Orange Soda, 12 oz.	151	37.6	0.0	99.6
Total	**1105**	**174.9**	**24.0**	**63.3**

MacDonald's Lunch or Dinner

	Energy (kcal)	CHO (grams)	Fat (% of Energy)	CHO (% of Energy)
Plain Hamburger with ketchup, 2	520	61.2	32.9	47.1
French Fries, regular serving	220	25.6	49.1	46.5
Hot Fudge Sundae, 1 each	284	47.7	31.2	67.2
Vanilla Milkshake, lowfat	290	60.0	3.1	82.8
Total	**1314**	**194.5**	**28.6**	**59.1**

Recommendations for Selecting High CHO Foods at Restaurants

PLACING AN ORDER

◆ Order a clear soup, tomato juice or V8 juice, steamed seafood, or fruit for an appetizer.

◆ Order a green salad with light dressing on the side. Avoid salads with cheese, eggs, meat, bacon or croutons. Avoid cole slaw or potato salad.

◆ Order broiled, roasted or baked lean meat, poultry or fish - even if the menu does not say broiled. Avoid casseroles and foods with heavy sauces.

◆ Order baked potato or plain rice - not pasta with sauces or fried or delmonico potatoes.

◆ Do not order dessert until you have eaten your main course. If you are still hungry, order sorbet, sherbet, frozen yogurt, ice milk, fruit or angel cake.

◆ Order juices - they are high in carbohydrates.

DURING THE MEAL

◆ Eat a plain roll, breadsticks or plain crackers rather than biscuits or croissants. Try to avoid spreads completely or use sparingly.

◆ Minimize your nibbling on nuts, buttery crackers, potato and tortilla chips.

◆ Ask the waiter to serve your salad immediately; use the dressing sparingly.

◆ Trim all visible fat off meat.

◆ Limit portions of margarine, butter or sour cream.

◆ Moderate your intake of alcoholic beverages.

Worksheet 8-1. Your Eating Out Checklist

Answer the following questions to see how many foods and food groups your meals usually include. THE MORE OFTEN YOU EAT THESE FOODS, THE HEALTHIER YOUR MEALS ARE.

How Often Does Your Lunch or Dinner Contain	Seldom or Never	1 or 2 Times per Week	3 or 4 Times per Week	Almost Daily
Fruits or fruit juices?	☐	☐	☐	☐
Vegetables or vegetable juices?	☐	☐	☐	☐
Enriched breads, pastas, or other grains?	☐	☐	☐	☐
Lean meat, fish, or poultry?	☐	☐	☐	☐
Beans, peas, lentils, tofu, nuts, or eggs?	☐	☐	☐	☐
Lowfat milk, cheese or yogurt?	☐	☐	☐	☐

Chapter 9
Nutritional Considerations For Endurance Activities

As SEALs you must be in excellent physical condition and be able to endure arduous physical tasks for extended periods of time. Your capacity to endure can be greatly improved by regular physical conditioning and by following special dietary practices. Prolonged running, swimming, load carrying and/or multiple shorter bouts of higher intensity activity impose significant demands on energy stores and fluid balance. Failure to replace the energy or fluids lost during prolonged operational or training activities can greatly impair your performance in subsequent mission activities. Meeting daily vitamin and mineral needs is also important since these micronutrients play an important part in physical performance (see Chapter 3). In this chapter, information on dietary interventions to enhance endurance performance is provided. It is important to remember that your daily energy intakes will vary according to your activity level.

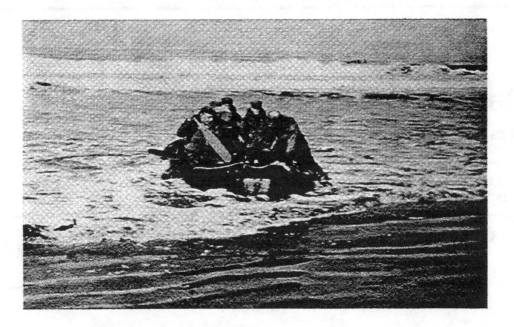

Glycogen Stores and Meeting Your Energy Needs

During heavy physical training you must increase your caloric intake especially from carbohydrate (CHO) foods to meet your energy demands. Failure to do so may result in:

◆ Chronic muscular fatigue

◆ A feeling of staleness

◆ Weight loss

◆ Poor sleep patterns

Liver and muscle glycogen is the primary source of glucose for your muscles during prolonged endurance activities. Therefore, the key to optimal endurance performance lies in maintaining muscle and liver glycogen stores. Once glycogen stores are exhausted, your ability to continue to perform an endurance activity will decrease sharply. When you wake up in the morning, your liver stores are low from not eating for several hours, and your blood glucose may be low. Thus, breakfast is critical to maintaining energy balance and liver glycogen stores.

> ## Keep a weight chart during periods of heavy training and arduous operations to document energy needs

Carbohydrates and Endurance Performance

Liver and muscle glycogen stores are replenished by eating carbohydrate (CHO) foods. Therefore:

> ## CHO is the most important energy-providing nutrient for endurance training

The endurance capacity of an individual on a high CHO diet is approximately three times greater than when on a high fat diet. When CHO intake is low, rigorous training sessions over several days will result in a gradual depletion of muscle glycogen stores and eventually impair performance. The figure below illustrates depletion of muscle glycogen over three days of running two hours per day. Note that when subjects ate a low CHO diet, glycogen stores gradually became depleted over the three day period. When the high CHO diet was consumed, glycogen stores were repleted between training sessions. Remember that glycogen is composed of glucose molecules linked together. This figure clearly demonstrates the need to consume foods that are high in CHO.

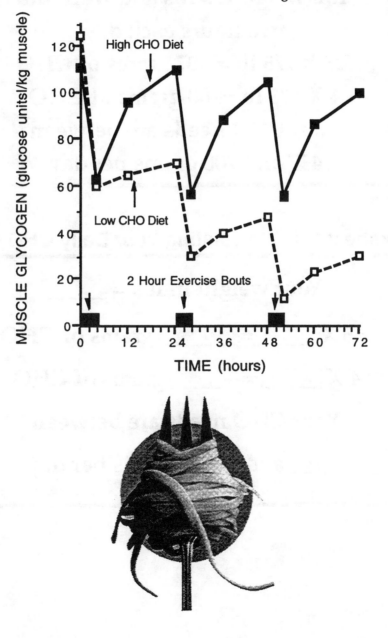

You should eat 2.5 to 4 grams CHO per pound of body weight each day.

EXAMPLE
You weigh 175 lbs and work out

two hours each day

2.5 X 175 lb = 437 grams of CHO

4 X 175 lb =700 grams of CHO

Your CHO needs are between

437 and 700 grams per day

Worksheet 9-1. Calculating Your Daily CHO Needs

Your weight in lbs = _____

2.5 X _____ = _____ grams of CHO

4 X _____ = _____ grams of CHO

Your CHO needs are between

_____ and _____ grams per day

Another way to think about CHO needs is in terms of energy intake. Ideally, *60 to 65%* of your daily energy should come from CHO. When energy intake is greater than 4,000 kcals then 60% is the proportion of CHO kcals to strive for. Since each gram of CHO is 4 kcal we can calculate the number of grams needed from your energy intake.

Example

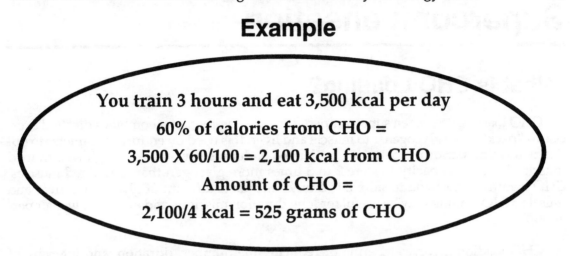

You train 3 hours and eat 3,500 kcal per day

60% of calories from CHO =

3,500 X 60/100 = 2,100 kcal from CHO

Amount of CHO =

2,100/4 kcal = 525 grams of CHO

List of various high CHO foods and the grams of CHO provided by each food is provided in Chapters 7 and 12 and Appendix 1. Complex CHO foods are preferable since they also provide vitamins and minerals in addition to CHO (see Chapter 2). Other important recommendations include:

Eat high CHO snacks in between training sessions to replace your glycogen stores.

Consume at least 50 grams of CHO immediately after completing your training session.

For example, you could eat a banana and drink a cup of orange juice. Commercially available high CHO liquid supplements may be beneficial during recovery from long training sessions because they supply CHO, water, protein, vitamins and minerals.

Keep a log of all CHO foods eaten for several days to see if your intake is high enough.

CHO Loading/ Glycogen Supercompensation

What is CHO Loading?

CHO loading/glycogen supercompensation is a regimen that combines diet and exercise to "pack" more glycogen into muscle and liver. It is used by endurance athletes to optimize physical performance during prolonged endurance events. Although well-trained muscles have the capacity to store 2 to 3 times more glycogen than untrained muscles, CHO loading allows you to store 2 to 4 times the usual amount of glycogen in liver and muscle. CHO loading may be useful for long duration missions and extended water operations.

CHO loading involves tapering or reducing the number, duration, and intensity of your training sessions the week prior to an event. As shown in the figure below, 5 days before the event (on day 2), be it an extended dive, land and water mission, or a sports competition, your training is tapered such that on days 2 and 3, no more than 40 minutes is spent on physical activities (solid line). CHO intake (dotted line) would be approximately 50% of your total energy intake. On days 4 and 5 the time spent exercising should be no more than 20 minutes, and your CHO intake should be increased to 70% of the total energy intake. Note day 6 is a rest day and CHO intake remains at 70% of the energy intake.

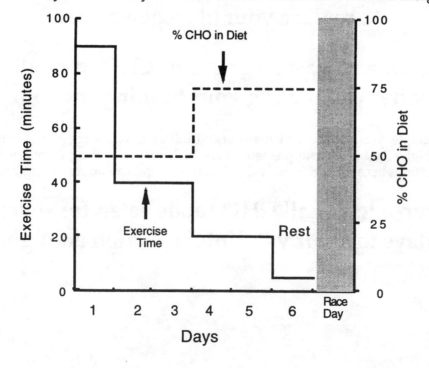

An accurate body weight should be obtained for reference purposes prior to modifying CHO intake and decreasing the intensity of training because 2.7 grams of water are stored with every gram of glycogen. Thus, on the day of the competition, if an additional 200 grams of glycogen have been stored, body weight should have increased by 0.54 kg or 1.2 pounds.

Who Should (and shouldn't) CHO Load?

For most regimens of intense physical training, a daily diet that provides 2.5 to 4 grams of CHO/lb body weight and adequate calories is sufficient to maintain muscle and liver glycogen reserves. However, for SDV operations, extended load-bearing marches, and other training scenarios with extremely high energy demands, CHO loading may prove to be very useful. Remember that CHO loading is not useful for events lasting only 60 minutes or less, and may in fact impair performance in activities requiring short bouts of maximal effort as you will weigh more from the additional water stored.

Protein Needs

Endurance training increases protein needs, and to meet the increased needs:

Protein intakes should range from 0.6 to 0.8 grams per pound body weight per day.

You calculated your protein requirements in Chapter 2 so refer back to that chapter for more information. It is likely your regular diet provides what you need because rarely do American men have protein intakes below the recommendations. Most men, including athletes, typically consume protein in excess of their actual needs.

Vitamin and Mineral Needs

Currently, the micronutrient requirements of people engaged in endurance activities are not well-defined. Because of the nature of your training, your daily overall needs may be 1.5 to 3 times greater than those of the average man. If you eat a healthy diet, your daily vitamin and mineral needs should be met from a variety of different foods (See Appendixes 5 and 6 for information on food sources of various vitamins and minerals). Because endurance exercise may increase your need for antioxidants, it is recommended that each day you should eat several foods rich in antioxidants (vitamin C, vitamin E and beta carotene), as shown in the table on the next page.

Table 9-1. Some Good Food Sources of Selected Antioxidant Nutrients

Vitamin C	Vitamin E	Beta Carotene
Orange juice	Sunflower seeds	Carrots
Grapefruit juice	Almonds	Spinach
Broccoli	Peanuts	Cantaloupe
Orange	Spinach	Broccoli
Strawberries	Olive oil	Winter squash
Cauliflower	Tomato	Dried apricots

Pay close attention to your electrolyte (sodium and potassium) needs when training in hot weather. You should get more than enough sodium in the foods you eat, whereas potassium requires a more careful selection of foods. See Appendix 6 for good food sources of potassium.

Fluid Requirements

Ingesting fluids at regular intervals and eating foods with a high water content are important for maintaining hydration and fluid status during training. Chapter 6 provides a thorough overview of fluid requirements and different types of beverages. In general:

Drink 1-2 cups of water 60 minutes before a training session.

Drink a cup of 5-8% CHO drink every 30 minutes during prolonged exercise.

During exercise, do not drink anything with a CHO content greater than 8% or you are likely to get stomach cramps.

Commercial fluid replacement beverages or diluted juices are recommended.

Consume beverages with a higher percentage (>8%) of CHO after exercise to replace glycogen stores and fluids lost during exercise.

The beverages you drink during and after prolonged exercise should contain sodium and potassium.

Nutritional Interventions During Training Sessions

Nutritional manipulations/interventions can delay fatigue and prevent conditions such as low blood sugar, dehydration, and low blood sodium that are detrimental to performance. These interventions include:

> **Drink 1 to 2 cups of a beverage supplemented with CHO (5 - 8%) and electrolytes every 30 minutes throughout exercise to extend your endurance.**

When an activity has been maintained for 2 to 3 hours without a CHO source, blood glucose levels may fall and cause fatigue. Ingestion of CHO beverages will prevent the fall in blood sugar (glucose) and delay fatigue. Although providing a CHO beverage 15 to 30 minutes before the anticipated onset of fatigue may extend performance for a short time, ingesting CHO after exhaustion will not allow you to immediately resume your activities.

> ## Consume CHO beverages at regular intervals during prolonged exercise.

Solid CHO foods, such as fruits and sports bars, are acceptable as CHO sources provided you are able to tolerate them during the activity and drink fluids with them. Food selections are personal choices and dietary manipulations should be tested during training and omitted if they prove troublesome to you. Some foods may cause stomach cramps and diarrhea if eaten during exercise. Dietary fiber intake should be limited during exercise to avoid gastrointestinal problems.

Summary

◆ Maintain energy balance by repleting glycogen stores between training sessions.

◆ Eat at least 2.5 grams of CHO per lb body weight or at least 400 grams of CHO per day to maintain your glycogen stores.

◆ Maximize glycogen stores before an event by ingesting 4 to 5 grams of CHO per lb body weight (or 70% of calories from CHO) for 2 to 3 days before the event.

◆ Drink at least 250 to 300 ml of a CHO supplemented (5-8%) beverage containing electrolytes every 30 minutes throughout prolonged training sessions.

◆ Consume at least 50 grams of CHO within 30 minutes of completing an extended training session and continue to eat/snack on high CHO foods every 2 hours for at least 6 hours to rapidly replace your glycogen stores.

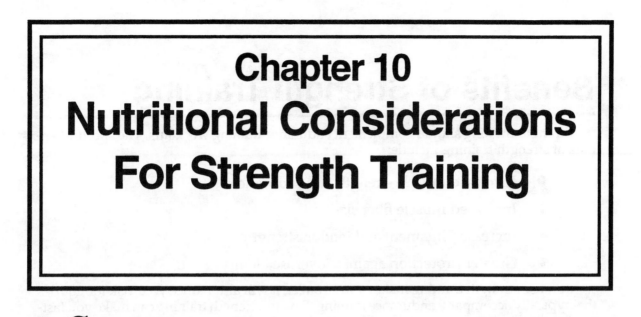

Chapter 10
Nutritional Considerations For Strength Training

*S*EAL missions and training require strength. Thus, a strength training program will enhance your physical conditioning and ability to perform and complete strenuous mission tasks. In addition, it will keep you "looking" fit! In this chapter information on strength training and the unique dietary requirements for strength training will be provided.

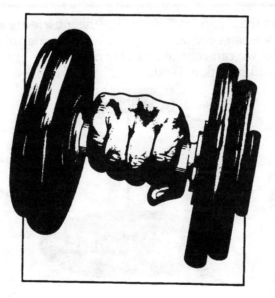

Benefits of Strength Training

Strength training should complement endurance training workouts. The specific benefits of strength training include:

- ◆ Increased muscle strength and endurance
- ◆ Increased muscle fiber size
- ◆ Increased ligament and tendon strength
- ◆ Greater protection against "overuse" injury

Because strength training makes you stronger, it will also reduce your risk for injuries that typically accompany endurance training. Finally, strength training can make you faster at tasks that require quick, short bursts of activity (such as a running from a boat to land).

Factors Determining Muscle Mass

The various factors that "regulate" the size of the muscle are shown below. Some, factors such as genetics, we can't control. Often we have no control over environmental factors either. Factors that we can control and play major roles in determining muscle mass are physical exercise and nutritional status.

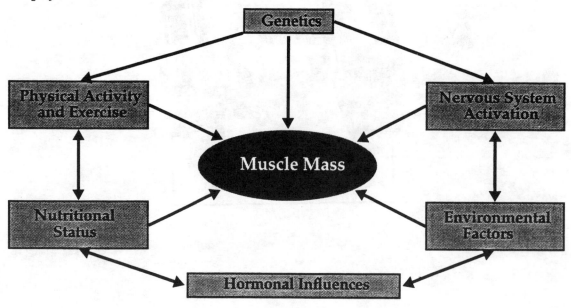

Protein Requirements For Strength Training

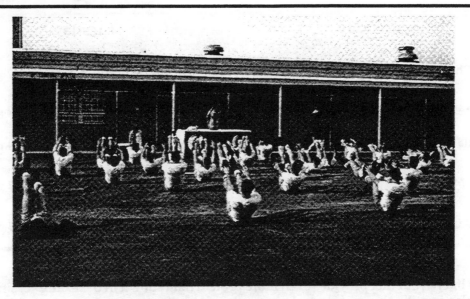

Research has shown that the protein needs of strength athletes and endurance athletes are quite similar: *You should eat 0.6 to 0.8 grams of protein per pound body weight each day to meet your daily protein requirements.*

Worksheet 10-1. How Much Protein Do I Need?

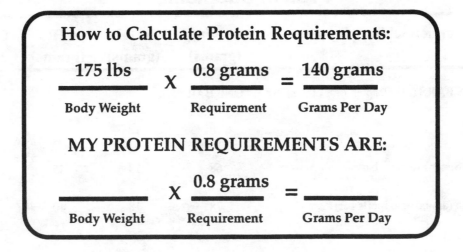

Table 10-1. Examples of Where You Get Protein

Monday		Tuesday	
8 oz Chicken Breast	72 grams	8 oz Broiled Sirloin Steak	62 grams
Subway Roast Beef Sandwich	41 grams	Subway Turkey Sandwich	42 grams
Vanilla Milkshake	9 grams	8 oz Bowl of Chili	19 grams
1 Egg McMuffin	18 grams	1 Sports Bar	12 grams
TOTAL	138 grams	TOTAL	135 grams

It is likely your diet provides even more protein than shown in the example, since protein is also in milk, cheese, fish, and many other foods. Some of you may be getting additional protein from commercially available sports bars, protein powders or carbohydrate/protein supplements as well as the foods you eat. Commercial supplements often provide considerable protein, as shown in the next table.

Table 10-2. Protein Content of Some Commercial Protein Supplements

Commercial Supplement	Serving (grams)	Protein (grams)	CHO (grams)	Calories/ Serving
SPORTS BARS (see Chapter 7 for others)	ONE BAR			
Hardbody	78	18	45	320
ICO Pro Super Protein™ bar	68	13	45	250
Oroamino (amino acid sports bar)	78	18	40	296

Table 10-2. Protein Content of Some Commercial Protein Supplements

Commercial Supplement	Serving (grams)	Protein (grams)	CHO (grams)	Calories/ Serving
BEVERAGES[1]				
Anabolic activator II	90	60	20	338
Bavarian Chocolate Cutting Advantage	65	25	37	225
Champion Nutrition Metabolol II™ (the meta-bolic optimizer)	66	17	42	260
Cybergenics Super Infiniti 3000	555	125	370	2400
Exceed Sports Meal	240	14	54	360
Hot Stuff (Advanced formula)	90	60	13	320
Joe Weider's Dynamic Muscle Builder	44	18	27	190
Joe Weider's Performance Muscle Builder	55	18	31	200
Mega Mass 2000	140	27	106	550
Met-Rx	72	37	24	262
Optimum Nutrition Mighty 1 3000	224	22	153	700
Twin Lab Opti Fuel 2	140	20	100	480
Twin Lab Anabolic Pre-Exercise Energy Drink. Mass Fuel	183	15	150	660
Victory Anabolic Cuts (low fat body definition mix)	42	15	24	170

[1]Beverage information is based on reconstituting one serving with water according to the manufacturer's directions. If these beverages were reconstituted with milk, calories and protein content would be higher.

The High Protein Myth

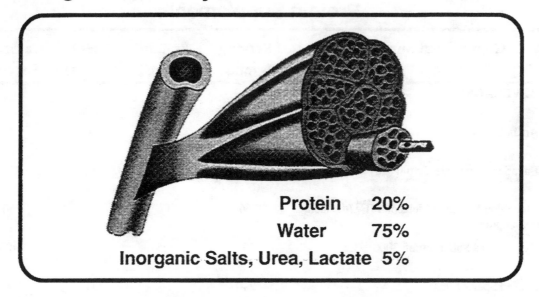

Protein	20%
Water	75%
Inorganic Salts, Urea, Lactate	5%

The excess protein in an athlete's diet, not required by the body, is often around 100 grams per day. Because muscle is 20% protein, the additional 100 grams of protein per day should result in a gain of 500 grams of muscle per day

Or about 1 pound of muscle per day.

If we look at what muscle is actually made up of we see that eating a high protein diet just doesn't add up. Muscle is only 20% protein; the rest is water and minerals, lactic acid, urea and high-energy phosphates.

If you ate 100 extra grams of protein every day for one week, you should gain 7 pounds of muscle mass! CLEARLY, this is not the case.

The extra protein results in an increase in the formation and excretion of the waste product "urea"; increases your fluid requirements; and places a considerable load on the liver and the kidneys.

You should avoid protein supplements that provide excessive amounts of protein or selected amino acids. Although heavily advertised, and in some cases endorsed by celebrities, very high protein intakes from supplements are NOT needed to build muscle. This practice can be very expensive, dangerous to your health, and quite unnecessary. A regular balanced diet can meet your protein needs very effectively.

Concerns With Very High Protein Intakes

◆ Increases the work load of the kidneys and in extreme cases result in kidney failure. In some individuals this practice has resulted in hypertension.

◆ Can be dehydrating especially during endurance events if additional fluids are not consumed.

◆ High intake of free amino acids may cause diarrhea and abdominal cramps.

◆ Creates imbalances of the essential amino acids.

Worksheet 10-2. How Much Protein Do I Eat?

For each weekday day over a one week period, write down all foods you ate that day that are high in protein. Using food labels and protein values in Appendix 3, record the protein content of each food in grams. For example: if you ate a hard-boiled egg and drank a glass of skim milk for breakfast on Monday, record under Monday those foods in the column labeled FOOD and in the column labeled G for grams enter 6 and 8. Similarly write down the food or protein supplement and its protein content for each day. Then, add up the numbers to see how many grams of protein you typically eat.

Monday		Tuesday		Wednesday		Thursday		Friday	
Food	G	Food	G	Food	G	Food	G	Food	G
TOTAL		TOTAL		TOTAL		TOTAL		TOTAL	

As you can see it is relatively easy to meet your daily protein requirements from food. You will probably find that your intake is far greater than your actual requirement.

Other Nutritional Requirements

Carbohydrate Requirements

Strength training relies on glycogen stores for energy. Thus, carbohydrates (CHO) are very important.

> ### 55 to 60% of your daily energy intake should come from CHO

The CHO recommendations for strength training are somewhat less than for endurance athletes since the overall energy requirements of weight lifting are less. BUT depending on your training schedule and length of your aerobic workouts, you may need 2.5 to 4 grams of CHO per pound body weight per day. For more information on carbohydrates see Chapters 2 and 9.

You may remember the term carbohydrate loading from Chapter 9. This practice is discouraged for weight lifters because of the extra water stored in the muscle. In other words, CHO loading provides no additional advantage in increasing muscle girth.

Fat Requirements

A thorough discussion of fat was provided in Chapter 2. But for fats in general, the recommendation is:

> ### Less than 30% of your energy should come from fat

Remember there are three different types of fat: monounsaturated, polyunsaturated and saturated fats and each should provide less than 10% of the daily energy.

Vitamins and Minerals

Meet your daily energy needs from a variety of different foods, should enable you to easily meet you vitamin and mineral needs. See Appendixes 5 and 6 for information on food sources of various vitamins and minerals.

Multi-Ingredient Steroid Alternatives - The Bottom Line

Some supplements containing herbs, glandulars, minerals such as chromium or boron, and a number of other compounds are being marketed as "muscle builders". Manufacturers claim that these products are *alternatives to steroids*. The major concerns associated with using such products are:

Not properly tested and absolutely no basis to substantiate the claims.

Potential for harmful side-effects, allergic reactions and toxicities.

Metabolic pathways and waste products formed from some of these compounds are not known.

Potential for testing positive for banned substances when using such products, especially those that do not reveal their "secret" ingredients.

Expensive and unlikely to replace the benefits of a good diet and sound training program.

If a product sounds too good to be true, it is usually not worth trying. Check Chapter 15 for more information on selected products or contact a sports nutritionist to verify the claims being made.

Summary

◆ Eat a wide variety of foods and match your energy intake to energy output.

◆ Aim for 0.6 and 0.8 grams of protein per pound per day or between 120 to 150 grams per day.

◆ Drink plenty of fluids.

◆ Don't get trapped into buying so called "muscle building" powders and potions. Proper training and a good diet will provide the lasting EDGE when it comes to building strength and muscles.

◆ SAVE YOUR MONEY or spend it on "real" foods.

Chapter 11
Nutrition for Optimum Mission Performance

*N*utrition is important for maximizing or optimizing mission performance. What you eat or don't eat before a physically demanding event could either "help" or "hurt" you. For example, eating a high fat meal before vigorous activity can slow you down as fat takes longer to digest than CHO. Knowing **when** to eat is also important since both fasting or eating a heavy meal shortly before endurance activity can decrease performance. Information to help optimize your performance during simulated and actual missions, including field deployment, is presented in this chapter. Suggestions for maximizing performance during BUDS training are also provided. In some instances you may be unable to control what or when you eat, however, it is important to meet your energy and fluid requirements.

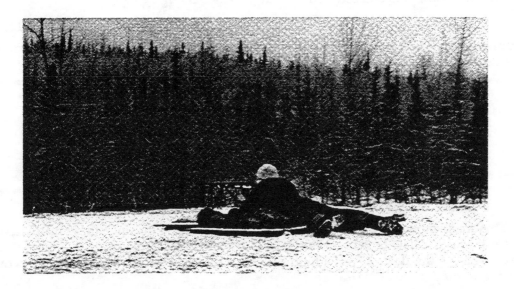

Nutritional Readiness Before a Specific Mission

In this scenario you may already be deployed under field conditions or locked down on base. Regardless of where you are, the two main considerations to nutritional readiness before missions are:

◆ Maximizing glycogen stores

◆ Being well-hydrated

In order to *be ready*, you must consider your pre-mission food and beverages.

Several Days Before a Mission

The average, lean, 175 pound man has approximately 1800 calories of carbohydrate (CHO) stored as glycogen in liver and muscle, and 75,000 to 150,000 calories stored as fat. In spite of these large energy stores in fat, once glycogen stores are exhausted, physical and mental performance will decrease and exhaustion will set in. A diet high in CHO for several days before a mission has the potential to increase liver and muscle glycogen stores, and thereby extend the time to exhaustion during a mission (see Chapter 9). Sample 3-day high CHO diet menus are provided in Appendix 7.

Timing and Composition of Pre-Mission Meals

A good pre-mission meal can increase glycogen stores in muscles and liver, and delay low blood sugar if it is correctly timed and provides enough CHO.

You should know your own tolerance for timing of meals and your ability to perform endurance activities. In general allow greater time for digestion before events that require intense physical activity.

> ### Eat up to 2 grams of CHO per pound body weight, but no more than 400 grams, 3 to 4 hours before a sustained operation.

This meal should provide a minimum of fat and protein, since these nutrients take longer to digest. CHO beverages and CHO/ protein drinks are excellent choices if taken 4 hours before the start. Avoid a high protein meal since this can increase fluid requirements and may cause dehydration.

> ## If you weigh 175 pounds
> ## $2 \times 175 = 350$ grams of CHO
>
> *You may eat up to 350 grams of CHO*
> *for your pre-mission meal*

If this is not possible, eat a small high CHO meal 2-3 hours before your mission (400 -500 calories).

A CHO beverage 1-2 hours before a mission will leave the stomach faster than a solid meal.

Nutrition for Maintaining Performance During Training and Missions

Three major nutrition-related issues encountered in the field are

◆ Inadequate ration consumption

◆ Dehydration

◆ Gastrointestinal complaints

Inadequate Ration Consumption

One of the biggest problems with eating rations is that it gets boring. Monotony and lack of time to eat contribute to decreased ration intake and weight loss.

Weight loss in the field is common and may impair mental and physical performance.

Therefore, it is important that you continue to consume your daily field ration so you can continue to perform.

Eat at least part of each ration item to get all essential nutrients

Limit your use of non-issue food items as meal/ration substitutes since they may be lacking in several important nutrients. Use these items as snacks to supplement your daily rations. Also pack high carbohydrate items, such as crackers, dried fruits, trail mixes, sports bars, etc. (see Chapter 7 for snack ideas). Experiment beforehand to see what suits you best. If you are planning to use high CHO bars check the fat content because if the fat content is greater than 3 g/100 calories it slows down absorption and can cause cramps.

If possible, drink 25 to 60 g of CHO/hr to maintain blood glucose.

Dehydration

You will become dehydrated if sweat and urine losses are not replaced by drinking water and other beverages (see Chapters 6 and 14). Dehydration may occur at any temperature and even under conditions of low levels of physical activity. Mild dehydration can decrease appetite and cause lethargy. Moderate dehydration decreases work capacity and severe dehydration could be fatal as shown in the figure on the next page.

Effects of Dehydration on Body Functions

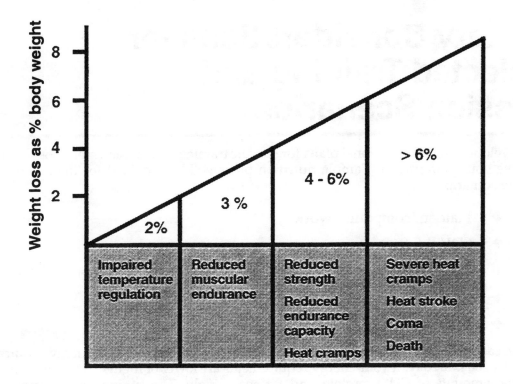

Drink water/fluids during water breaks.
You should drink at least 4 canteens per day, or
more if you are in a hot environment.

See Chapters 6 and 14 for more information on fluid replacement.

Monitor the color of your urine; if your urine is dark, increase fluid consumption until the color becomes pale yellow. If you are taking B vitamin supplements, your urine may not be pale but bright yellow.

Gastrointestinal Complaints

Change in diet, dehydration, too much fiber, poor sanitary conditions or stress may result in diarrhea or constipation in the field. Make sure you are well hydrated at all times, and avoid trying new non-issue foods unless they have passed sanitation inspection.

Dietary Considerations for Selected Training and Mission Scenarios

Developing sound nutritional plans for specific training and mission scenarios should improve your performance. Sample nutrition plans will be provided for the following training scenarios.

- ◆ Platoon/compound work

- ◆ SDV sub trips

- ◆ Typical land warfare

- ◆ Double dive days

- ◆ BUDS - Phases 1, 2 and 3

For each scenario, the macronutrient recommendation assumes an energy requirement of 4,000 kcal/day. If your energy requirements are lower or higher, you will need to alter the amounts of CHO, protein and fat accordingly. **The timing and/or nutrient amount at any particular time can be modified to suit your individual needs based on the scenario and your personal experiences.** Snacks refers to food and beverages that can be carried and consumed while on the go.

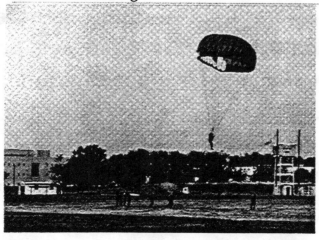

Table 11-1. Seal Team Platoon/Compound Work

This scenario requires small meals throughout the day to help maintain blood sugar and energy levels. Remember to drink fluids regularly.

	CHO	Protein (grams)	Fat
0530 - Wake up			
0600 - CHO/ prot beverage	50	10	-
0700-830 - Work out			
0830 - Breakfast	125	25	25
0900 - Start department/ Platoon work			
1000 - Snack	50	10	10
1130 - Break for lunch	125	30	35
1230 - Return for department/ Platoon work			
1400 - Snack	50	5	10
1600 - End work day			
1700 - Possible second work out			
1830-1900 - Dinner	150	30	35
2200 - Snack	50	10	10
TOTAL	600	120	125
% of 4000 calories	60%	12%	28%

Table 11-2. SDV Sub Trip

These maneuvers can cover 18 - 20 hours/day for several days; this makes recovery a crucial aspect of continued, optimal performance. Nutritional preparedness for this scenario includes replenishing glycogen stores and being well hydrated at all times.

	CHO	Protein (grams)	Fat
0700 - Breakfast	125	30	20
0830 - Rig Zodials for Sub Lock Out			
1000 - Snack	50	10	5
1200 - Lunch	125	30	20
1400 - Brief			
1600 - CHOW	125	25	15
1700 - Jock up			
1800 - Dive			
1900 - Begin Lock Out of Sub op to Beach			
2200 - CHO Beverage	50	10	5
2400 - Beverage	50	10	-
0200 - Beverage	50	10	-
0400 - Dive - Lock In			
0600 - De- jock/ Clean up			
0630 - Snack	75	25	25
TOTAL	650	150	90
% of 4000 calories	65%	15%	20%

Table 11-3. Typical Land Warfare

Typical land warfare operations can continue for 3 to 4 weeks, so it is important to avoid losing weight during this period. Eat CHO snacks with some protein when you feel drowsy (see Chapter 7 for snack ideas).

	CHO	Protein (grams)	Fat
0800 - (PT/ Breakfast) _____	125	20	15
0900 - Muster			
0930 - Range (Hot environment- 1600 Shooting and moving in combat gear)			
1030 - Snack _____	50	10	5
1200 - Lunch _____	125	20	20
1400 - Snack _____	50	10	5
1600 - Dinner/ rest _____	125	30	30
1900 - Snack _____	50	10	5
2100 - Range (Late night fire 2400 and movement)			
2200 - Snack _____	50	10	5
2400 - Cut loose			
2400 - Snack _____	75	10	15
2430 - Clean weapons			
TOTAL	650	120	100
% of 4000 calories	65%	12%	23%

Table 11-4. Double Dive Day (for 3 weeks)

Double dive day series which continue for 3 weeks require adequate recovery between dives. Water operations are associated with high energy expenditure and fluid losses, especially when in cold water (see Chapter 14).

	CHO	Protein (grams)	Fat
0600-CHO/prot beverage	50	10	-
0630-0800 - Physical training			
0800- Breakfast	100	20	5
0830-1000 - Classroom/dive prep			
1000-1200 - Dive			
1100- Snack	50	10	-
1200-1330 - Lunch	150	40	40
1330-1600 - Class/gear prep			
1430- Snack	50	10	5
1600-1730 - Dinner	75	20	15
1800-2400 - Brief dive, downstage			
2000-CHO/prot beverage	50	10	-
2200-CHO/prot beverage	50	10	-
2400- Snack	75	20	25
2400-0600 - Personal time			
TOTAL	650	150	90
% of 4000 calories	65%	15%	20%

Nutrition for Optimum Mission Performance

Table 11-5. Typical BUDs Training Day- 1st Phase

Phase I training at BUDs is grueling. Many trainees drop-out because they cannot manage the physical and psychological demands; eating to win may help them succeed. Importantly, the energy expended requires a matching energy input. Some suggestions for timing and distribution of energy are provided in this table.

	CHO	Protein (grams)	Fat
0600-0730 - Breakfast	100	15	10
0745-0930 - Obstacle Course			
0930-CHO/prot beverage	50	10	-
0930-1030 - Classroom			
1030-1130 - Conditioning run			
1130-1300 Lunch	150	40	40
1300-1330 - Classroom - Dive Brief			
1330-1600 - 1 mile Bay Swim without Fins			
1600-1800 - Dinner	150	40	45
2000-2100- Snack	100	15	25
2200-CHO/prot beverage	50	10	-
TOTAL	600	130	120
% of 4000 calories	60%	13%	27%

Table 11-6. Typical BUDs Training Day - 2nd Phase

Phase 2 training which involves multiple bouts of physical activity each day makes recovery between bouts an important aspect of optimizing physical performance. Make sure you are well hydrated at all times.

	CHO	Protein (grams)	Fat
0600-0730 - Breakfast	100	20	15
0730-0800 - Pre-Dive			
0800-CHO/ prot beverage	50	10	-
0800-0900 - Dive Brief			
0900-1130 - Dive			
1130-CHO/ prot beverage	50	10	-
1130-1300 - Lunch	125	40	40
1300-1430 - Post/Pre-Dive			
1430-1630 - PT-Run	50	10	5
1630-1800 - Dinner	125	20	25
1800-1900 - Dive Brief			
1900-2130- Dive			
2130-CHO/prot beverage	100	20	-
2130-2230 - Post Dive			
2230-Snack	75	20	25
TOTAL	600	150	110
% of 4000 calories	60%	15%	25%

Table 11-7. Typical BUDs Training Day- 3rd Phase

In this situation you would want to eat a light lunch to avoid feeling uncomfortable during the 6 mile run. Instead, drink a CHO containing beverage or eat a high CHO snack (see Chapter 7) while at the pistol range. As in every scenario, here too it is important to be well hydrated at all times (see Chapter 6).

	CHO	Protein (grams)	Fat
0600-0700 - Breakfast	100	20	30
0700-1200 - Pistol Range			
0900-CHO/ prot beverage	50	10	-
1000-CHO/ prot beverage	50	10	-
1200-1300 - Lunch	100	20	15
1300-1500 -DEMO classroom			
1500-1600 - Conditioning run (6 miles)			
1600-CHO /protein beverage	100	20	-
1600-1630 - Transit locations			
1630-1730 - Dinner	125	45	45
1730-2000 - Review (classroom)			
2200-Snack	75	25	20
TOTAL	600	150	110
% of 4000 calories	60%	15%	25%

Other Considerations

For all of the sample scenarios, the following recommendations apply:

◆ Eat a variety of foods

◆ Maintain energy balance

◆ Maintain hydration status

◆ Include high CHO snacks in between meals to replenish/maximize glycogen stores (especially if there are two periods of high activity)

◆ See Chapter 14 for additional considerations about training or operating in the heat, cold, and other adverse conditions.

Dietary Composition

The breakdown of energy from CHO, protein and fat should be 60 to 65% from CHO, 10 to 15% from protein, and 20 to 30% from fat. When energy requirements are above 4000 kcal, more fat may be required since it is difficult to get sufficient calories from CHO alone. Recommendations for the approximate gram amounts of CHO, protein, and fat for various energy levels are shown in the following table.

Table 11-8. Recommended Grams of CHO, Protein and Fat for Various Energy Levels

Energy Level (kcal)	CHO (grams)	Protein (grams)	Fat (grams)
3000	500	110	65
3500	550	115	90
4000	650	125	100
4500	700	135	125
5000	700	160	170

Vitamins and Minerals

As of now there are no definitive recommendations. If you meet your energy requirements from a variety of foods, by including fruits and vegetables, you should be able to meet your vitamin and mineral requirements (see Appendixes 5 and 6). Selected recommendations would be to:

◆ Include foods that are good sources of antioxidants in your daily diet.

◆ If you feel you need to take vitamin and mineral supplements follow the guidelines presented in Chapter 4.

◆ During extended dive series you may want to consider taking a multi-mineral supplement.

Immersion in water, especially cold, can increase urinary losses of magnesium, calcium, zinc and chromium (see Chapter 4 for safe amounts).

Fluid and Electrolytes

All of the scenarios require adequate fluids. Immersion increases fluid losses and operations in a warm/hot environment deplete body water. Replace electrolytes lost through sweating by consuming a fluid replacement beverage that contains electrolytes or by eating foods that contain these nutrients (see Chapter 12 and Appendix 6).

Forced drinking is highly recommended for all environments since normal thirst mechanisms cannot keep up with increased requirements. See Chapter 6 for the ideal composition of fluid replacement beverages.

Chapter 12
Nutritional Interventions for Mission Recovery

*A*fter a mission it is important that you recover quickly and continue to train and prepare for the next mission. A quick recovery will enhance preparedness, boost morale and help protect you from training injuries. Both rest and nutrition play an important part in the recovery process. In this chapter information about nutritional measures that can help you speed up your recovery after a mission is provided.

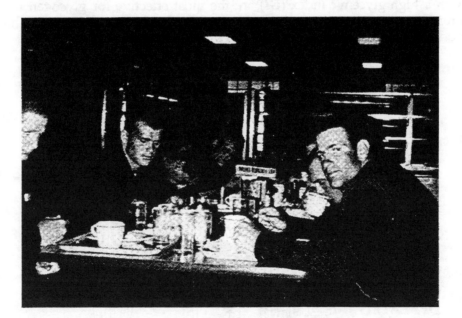

Glycogen Restoration

Glycogen depletion is common following prolonged events requiring sustained physical activity. For example, an extended dive, sustained efforts on land, and prolonged shivering can deplete muscle glycogen stores. During recovery it is critical that these stores be repleted, and nutritional interventions can accelerate the process.

Glycogen repletion in muscles takes place at a relatively constant rate as long as blood glucose remains elevated. In other words, blood glucose must be high for it to be made available to muscle for storage.

To optimize glycogen restoration consume 50 grams of carbohydrate (CHO) soon after the completion of the mission, and 50 grams of CHO every two hours for six hours after the mission.

Ingestion of greater amounts of CHO will not further increase the rate of glycogen resynthesis.

Not all CHO foods are equally effective in restoring glucose. Certain foods are better at raising blood glucose concentrations and promoting glycogen synthesis. The term *Glycemic Index* is used to describe how high a particular food will raise blood glucose levels; foods with a high glycemic index (*GI*) are the most effective for glycogen restoration. Thus, after a mission, consume foods and beverages that have a moderate to high *GI*. A list of foods classified according to their *GI* is provided on the next page.

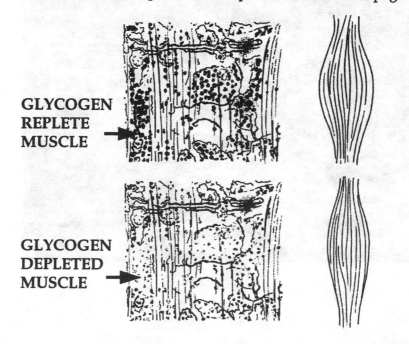

GLYCOGEN REPLETE MUSCLE

GLYCOGEN DEPLETED MUSCLE

Table 12-1. A Selection of Foods with a High, Moderate, or Low Glycemic Index

Foods	Amount of Food Required for 50 grams of CHO
Highly Glycemic Foods	
Bagel	1.3 bagel
Bread (white or whole wheat)	4.2 slices
Cornflakes	2.5 cups
Honey	2.9 tbsp
Maple syrup	3.1 tbsp
Potato, baked w/ skin	1 medium
Raisins	0.4 cup
Shredded Wheat Cereal	1.4 cups
Sweet Corn, cooked	1.5 cups
Watermelon	4.5 cups
Moderately Glycemic Foods	
Baked Beans	1.0 cup
Banana	1.8 medium
Grapes	55 grapes
Oatmeal, cooked	2.0 cups
Orange Juice	2.0 cups
Rice, cooked	1 cup
Sweet Potato, boiled	0.8 cup

Foods	Amount of Food Required for 50 grams of CHO
Low Glycemic Foods	
Apple	2.5 medium
Peaches	5 medium
Pear	2 medium
Green Peas, cooked	2.2 cups
Ice Cream	1.6 cups
Spaghetti and Other Pasta, cooked	1.4 cups
Yogurt, nonfat plain	2.9 cups

Rehydration

Begin rehydrating immediately after the mission.

After a mission, forced fluid ingestion is essential because the sensation of thirst may be blunted. **Typically, voluntary consumption of fluids will restore only half of the fluid lost.** If possible, weigh yourself after the mission and compare this weight to your usual weight. Over a period of several hours you should:

Drink at least two 8 oz. cups of fluid for every pound of body weight lost.

Fluid replacement beverages ingested during exercise are also appropriate for rehydration. Fluids used for rehydration after a mission can contain a higher percentage of CHO than those used during exercise. A list of various fluid replacement beverages and more information on fluid replacement techniques is provided in Chapter 6.

Sodium/Electrolyte Replacement

Sodium and potassium losses in sweat can be quite high during prolonged physical activity, especially in warm weather. Replacing these electrolytes is an important part of the recovery process. Most commercially available fluid replacement beverages contain electrolytes. Also, sodium is widely present in a variety of foods, but if the weather is warm:

Each quart of fluid should contain about one quarter teaspoon of salt.

A little bit of salt will speed up rehydration better than plain water. Typically, commercial fluid replacement beverages contain both sodium and potassium, but your recovery foods should also include foods rich in potassium. Some excellent food sources of potassium are listed below and additional information is provided in Appendix 6. You will notice that these foods are also good sources of CHO and most have a moderate to high glycemic index.

Table 12-2. Good Sources Of Potassium

Foods	Beverages
Banana	Orange juice
Apricots, dried	Tomato juice
Dates	Pineapple juice
Dried peaches	Grapefruit juice
Melons	Skim Milk
Baked potato	
Yogurt	

NOTE: 1 cup of orange juice or tomato juice will replace the potassium, calcium and magnesium lost in 3 quarts of sweat.

Summary

◆ High CHO foods and beverages are ideal recovery foods

◆ Consume 50 grams of CHO as food or drink immediately after mission completion and 50 grams every 2 hours for 6 hours

◆ Choose foods and drinks with a moderate to high glycemic index to accelerate glycogen repletion

◆ Drink plenty of fluids after a gruelling mission, even if you are not thirsty

◆ Your fluid replacement beverages should contain sodium and potassium

◆ Fruit juices are excellent recovery fluids as they provide CHO, vitamins, minerals, sodium and potassium

◆ If you can't tolerate solid foods after intense physical exertion, drink a CHO containing beverage (see chapters 6 and 9 for additional information on CHO containing beverages)

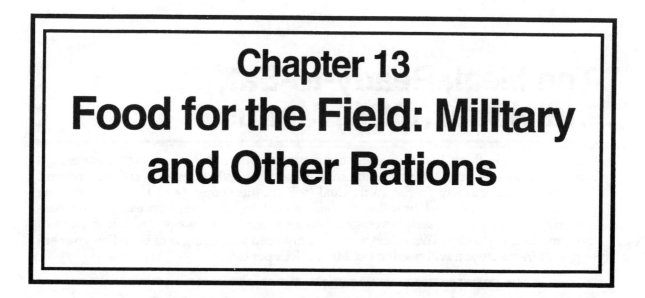

Chapter 13
Food for the Field: Military and Other Rations

*F*ield rations are designed to supply adequate energy and nutrients for a particular type of mission. Since the duration and environmental conditions of missions vary, different types of operational rations have been developed. For example, there are cold weather rations for frigid conditions, and light weight rations for missions lasting no longer than 30 days. These rations have different caloric contents with varying proportions of fat, protein, and carbohydrate to meet the nutritional demands of the various conditions. This chapter describes what rations are available and compares some military and commercially prepared foods. You can decide where your money would best be spent after comparing their distribution of calories.

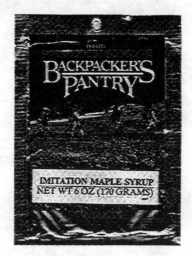

The Meal, Ready-to-Eat, Individual (MRE) Menus

Many people think that military rations are sub-optimal: Not enough calories, too much fat, bad taste, and too much salt are some claims leveled against military rations. The revised Meal, Ready-To-Eat, Individual (MRE) ration consists of 12 meals (see next page for menus); each meal, or menu, contains an entree, crackers, a spread (cheese, peanut butter, or jelly), a dessert, beverages, and an accessory package. No rehydration of these meals is necessary. This ration will certainly keep you going and based on your energy requirements you will need to eat 2 to 4 MREs per day.

> ## Each menu provides 1300 Calories
> ## 49% CHO, 15% protein, 36% fat
> ## Supplemental Bread Pouch: 200 Calories
> ## 55% CHO, 12% protein, 33% fat,

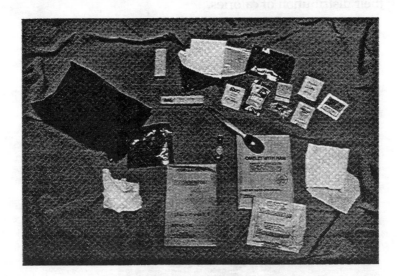

It is also important to note that some components of the MRE have been supplemented with selected vitamins (A, B_1, B_2, niacin, B_6, and C) and minerals (calcium). Fortified items include cocoa beverage powder, cheese spread, peanut butter, crackers, oatmeal cookies coating, and brownies coating.

Table 13-1. MRE Menus

MENU 1	MENU 2	MENU 3	MENU 4	MENU 5	MENU 6
Pork W/ Rice In BBQ Sauce	Corned Beef Hash	Chicken Stew	Omelet w/ Ham	Spaghetti w/ Meat & Sauce	Chicken A La King
Apple sauce[1]	Fruit[2]	Fruit[1]	Potato Au Gratin	Fruit[2]	
	Oatmeal Cookie Bar		Oatmeal Cookie Bar	Maple Nut Cake	
Jelly	Jelly	Peanut Butter	Cheese Spread	Cheese Spread	Peanut Butter
Crackers	Crackers	Crackers	Crackers	Crackers	Crackers
				Candy[3]	Candy[3]
Cocoa Beverage	Cocoa Beverage	Cocoa Beverage	Cocoa Beverage		Cocoa Beverage
Beverage Powder	Beverage Powder	Beverage Powder	Beverage Powder	Beverage Powder	Beverage Powder
Hot Sauce	Hot Sauce	Hot Sauce	Hot Sauce	Hot Sauce	Hot Sauce
Packet B	Packet B	Packet B	Packet B	Packet A	Packet A
Spoon	Spoon	Spoon	Spoon	Spoon	Spoon

MENU 7	MENU 8	MENU 9	MENU 10	MENU 11	MENU 12
Beef Stew	Ham Slice	Meatballs & Rice in Spicy Tomato Sauce	Tuna w/ Noodles	Chicken w/ Rice	Escalloped Potatoes w/ Ham
	Potato Au Gratin	Fruit[2]			Apple sauce[1]
Cherry Nut Cake	Brownie, Chocolate Covered	Cookie, Chocolate Covered	Chocolate Nut Cake	Cookie, Chocolate Covered	Brownie, Chocolate Covered
Peanut Butter	Jelly	Peanut Butter	Cheese Spread	Cheese Spread	Jelly
Crackers	Crackers	Crackers	Crackers	Crackers	Crackers
				Candy	Candy
	Cocoa Beverage				Cocoa Beverage
Beverage Powder	Beverage Powder	Beverage Powder	Beverage Powder	Beverage Powder	Beverage Powder
Hot Sauce	Hot Sauce	Hot Sauce	Hot Sauce	Hot Sauce	Hot Sauce
Packet A	Packet A	Packet A	Packet A	Packet A	Packet A
Spoon	Spoon	Spoon	Spoon	Spoon	Spoon

Packet A: Coffee, Cream Substitute, Sugar, Salt, Chewing Gum, Matches, Toilet Tissue, Towelette

Packet B: Coffee, Cream Substitute, Sugar, Salt, Chewing Gum, Matches, Toilet Tissue, Towelette, Candy (Vanilla Caramels, Tootsie Rolls, or Heat Stable Chocolate Bar)

[1]Thermostablized: [2]Freeze-Dried Fruit: Peaches, Pears, Fruit Mix, or Strawberries

[3]Charms or Heat Stable M&M's

Ration, Cold Weather (RCW)

The Ration, Cold Weather (RCW) was designed to sustain individuals during operations in cold conditions. The six menus should provide sufficient calories to meet energy requirements during strenuous exercises in extreme cold. The ration is high in carbohydrate (CHO) since this macronutrient generates more heat, and comes as two meal bags, Bag A and Bag B. Each menu is sufficient for a 24 hour period, but more can be eaten when energy needs are higher. The RCW is also lower in salt and protein than the MREs to reduce daily water requirements and lessen the possibility of dehydration. If consumed hydrated, one day's ration requires 90 ounces (about 9 cups or 3 canteens) of water. Although it could get very boring, it will definitely help maintain your performance.

> ## Each menu provides 4500 Calories
> ## 60% CHO, 8% protein, 32% fat
> ## Sodium content: 5 grams

Table 13-2. Ration, Cold Weather Menus

	MENU 1	MENU 2	MENU 3	MENU 4	MENU 5	MENU 6
BAG A	Oatmeal, Strawberry & Cream	Oatmeal, Apple & Cinnamon	Oatmeal, Apple & Cinnamon	Oatmeal, Maple & Brown Sugar	Oatmeal, Strawberry & Cream	Oatmeal, Maple & Brown Sugar
	Nut Raisin Mix	Nut Raisin Mix	Nut Raisin Mix	Nut Raisin Mix	Nut Raisin Mix	Nut Raisin Mix
	Cocoa Beverage Powder (2)	Cocoa Beverage Powder (2)	Cocoa Beverage Powder (2)	Cocoa Beverage Powder (2)	Cocoa Beverage Powder (2)	Cocoa Beverage Powder (2)
	Apple Cider Mix	Apple Cider Mix	Apple Cider Mix	Apple Cider Mix	Apple Cider Mix	Apple Cider Mix
	Chicken Noodle Soup	Chicken Noodle Soup	Chicken Noodle Soup	Chicken Noodle Soup	Chicken Noodle Soup	Chicken Noodle Soup
	Fruit Bars, (Fig or Blueberry)	Fruit Bars, (Fig or Blueberry)	Fruit Bars, (Fig or Blueberry)	Fruit Bars, (Fig or Blueberry)	Fruit Bars, (Fig or Blueberry)	Fruit Bars, (Fig or Blueberry)
	Crackers (2)	Crackers (2)	Crackers (2)	Crackers (2)	Crackers (2)	Crackers (2)
	Spoon	Spoon	Spoon	Spoon	Spoon	Spoon
	Accessory Packet	Accessory Packet	Accessory Packet	Accessory Packet	Accessory Packet	Accessory Packet

Table 13-2. Ration Cold Weather Menus

	MENU 1	MENU 2	MENU 3	MENU 4	MENU 5	MENU 6
BAG B	Chicken Stew	Beef Stew	Chili Con Carne	Chicken A La King	Chicken & Rice	Spaghetti w/ Meat Sauce
	Granola Bars (2)	Granola Bars (2)	Granola Bars (2)	Granola Bars (2)	Granola Bars (2)	Granola Bars (2)
	Oatmeal Cookie Bars (2)	Oatmeal Cookie Bars (2	Oatmeal Cookie Bars (2	Oatmeal Cookie Bars (2	Oatmeal Cookie Bars (2	Oatmeal Cookie Bars (2
	Chocolate Covered Cookie or Brownie	Chocolate Covered Cookie or Brownie	Chocolate Covered Cookie or Brownie	Chocolate Covered Cookie or Brownie	Chocolate Covered Cookie or Brownie	Chocolate Covered Cookie or Brownie
	Orange Beverage Powder	Orange Beverage Powder	Orange Beverage Powder	Orange Beverage Powder	Orange Beverage Powder	Orange Beverage Powder
	Tootsie Rolls	Tootsie Rolls	Tootsie Rolls	Tootsie Rolls	Tootsie Rolls	Tootsie Rolls
	M&M's	M&M's	M&M's	M&M's	M&M's	M&M's
	Lemon Tea (2)	Lemon Tea (2)	Lemon Tea (2)	Lemon Tea (2)	Lemon Tea (2)	Lemon Tea (2)
	Spoon	Spoon	Spoon	Spoon	Spoon	Spoon

Accessory Packet: Coffee, Cream, Sugar, Chewing Gum, Toilet Paper (2), Matches, Closure Device (2)

Ration Lightweight - 30 Days (RLW-30)

This ration was designed for individuals of the Special Operation Forces who might participate in reconnaissance missions of up to 30 days. Thus, it is as it's name: a low weight, low volume ration. There are six menus, each consisting of dehydrated, compressed, and "low water containing" foods. The foods may be eaten dry or reconstituted with water.

> ## Each menu provides 2132 Calories
> ## 52% CHO, 18% protein, 30% fat
> ## Sodium content: 5 grams

If this ration is used during extended operations, more CHO would be needed to obtain the recommended amount (at least 400 grams); it provides only 277 grams as is.

Table 13-3. Ration Lightweight Menus

MENU 1	MENU 2	MENU 3	MENU 4	MENU 5	MENU 6
Chicken A La King	Beef Stew	Pork with Rice	Chicken w/ Rice & Ham	Spaghetti with Meat & Sauce	Chili Con Carne
Cheese Bread Crisp	Tamale Bread Crisp	Pizza Bread Crisp	Cheese-Bacon Bread Crisp	Coconut Bread Crisp	Orange-Nut Bread Crisp
Almond Dairy Bar	Strawberry Dairy Bar	Pecan Dairy Bar	Orange Cream-sicle Dairy Bar	Mixed Nut Dairy Bar	Maple Walnut Dairy Bar
Blueberry Dessert Bar	Chocolate Chip Dessert Bar	Apple Cinnamon Dessert Bar	Pecan Dessert Bar	Chocolate Halva Dessert Bar	Graham Dessert Bar
Shredded Wheat Cereal Bar	Wheat Flake Cereal Bar	Bran Flake Cereal Bar	Oat Cereal Biscuit Bar	Malted Wheat Granules Cereal Bar	Corn Flakes Cereal Bar
Tropical Punch Bar	Lemonade Beverage Bar	Orange Beverage Bar	Lemon-Lime Beverage Bar	Strawberry Beverage Bar	Raspberry Beverage Bar
Cocoa Beverage Bar	Cocoa Beverage Bar	Cocoa Beverage Bar	Cocoa Beverage Bar	Cocoa Beverage Bar	Cocoa Beverage Bar
Beef Snacks	Beef Snacks	Beef Snacks	Beef Snacks	Beef Snacks	Beef Snacks

Accessory Packet (5/case): Instant Coffee (6), Cream Substitute (3), Sugar (3), Chewing Gum (6), Instant Tea (6), Matches (2), Toilet Tissue (6), Plastic Picnic Spoon (2), Closure Device (1).

Food Packet, Long Range Patrol, (Improved) (LRP[I])

This ration was designed for special operations and initial assaults and has a shelf life of 10 years. The eight menus, which have been revised significantly since the ration was used during the Vietnam war, consist of dehydrated entrees, cereal bars, candy and instant beverages. Each menu requires approximately 28 oz. of water to prepare, although some of the foods may be eaten dry. It is lightweight, has proven acceptance, and is relatively inexpensive.

Each LRP[I] menu provides 1570 Calories
50% CHO, 15% protein, 35% fat
Sodium content: 2.6 grams

To obtain adequate CHO and calories during extended operations, at least two menus would need to be eaten; one menu provides only 195 grams of CHO as is.

Table 13-4. Long Range Patrol (LRP[I])

MENU 1	MENU 2	MENU 3	MENU 4
Chicken Stew	Beef Stew	Escalloped Potato & Pork	Chicken in White Sauce w/ Vegetables
Cornflake Bar	Granola Bar	Cornflake & Rice Bar	Cornflake Bar
Oatmeal Cookie Bar	Chocolate Covered Cookie	Fig Bar	Chocolate Covered Cookie
Tootsie Rolls (4)	Caramels	Chocolate Bars w/ Toffee (2)	Chuckles
Apple Cider Drink	Cocoa Beverage	Apple Cider Drink	Orange Beverage
Spoon	Spoon	Spoon	Spoon
Accessory Packet	Accessory Packet	Accessory Packet	Accessory Packet

MENU 5	MENU 6	MENU 7	MENU 8
Chicken & Rice	Spaghetti w/ Meatsauce	Chili Con Carne	Beef & Rice
Granola Bar	Cornflake & Rice Bar	Granola Bar	Cornflake Bar
Chocolate Covered Brownie	Oatmeal Cookie Bar	Chocolate Covered Brownie	Fig Bar

Table 13-4. Long Range Patrol (LRP[I])

Chuckles	Tootsie Rolls (4)	Charms	M & M's
Lemon Tea (2)	Beverage Base (MRE)	Orange Beverage	Lemon Tea (2)
Accessory Packet	Accessory Packet	Accessory Packet	Accessory Packet
Spoon	Spoon	Spoon	Spoon

Accessory Packet: Coffee, Creamer, Sugar, Chewing Gum, Toilet Paper (2), Matches, Salt

Commercial Freeze-Dried Products

Light weight, freeze-dried foods are commercially available from a number of manufacturers. Two of the most popular manufacturers are Mountain House and AlpineAire. As with any food manufacturer, their products differ in terms of taste, caloric distribution, protein, and sodium content. Many of the items from both companies have been tested under field conditions for up to 30 days, and the acceptability varied from person to person. Choose a ration that will provide adequate calories and CHO to fit your requirements.

Table 13-5. Here's a Look at Two Similar Dinner Entrees From the Two Companies:

Menu: Chili

Macronutrients	Mountain House	AlpineAire
Total Calories	220	340
% Fat	25%	5%
% Protein	22%	28%
% CHO	55%	64%

Menu: Beef Stroganoff

Macronutrients	Mountain House	AlpineAire
Total Calories	250	306
% Fat	43%	18%
% Protein	14%	29%
% CHO	43%	59%

Note the differences in total calories and the distribution of calories. For example, Mountain House Beef Stroganoff provides 8.8 grams of protein whereas AlpineAire's Beef Stroganoff provides 22 grams. This shows how important it is to check the nutritional listing on the package label. A variety of other meals and their macronutrient distribution is provided on the following pages.

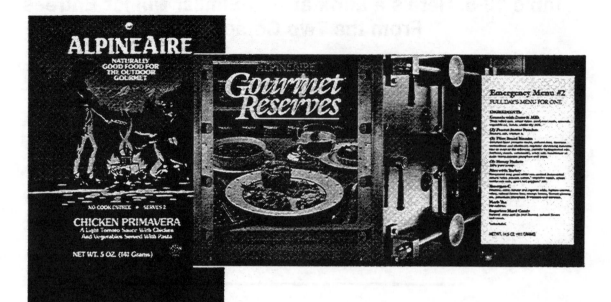

Table 13-6. Selected Foods and Menus From AlpineAire

Items	Serving Size	Calories per Serving	CHO (grams)	Protein (grams)	Fat (grams)	Sodium (mg)
ENTREES						
MOUNTAIN CHILI	3.5 OZ.	340	54	24	2	1,334
LEONARDO DA FETTUCINE	2.75 OZ.	295	45	15	3	686
CHEESE NUT CASSEROLE	3.25 OZ.	372	62	16	16	1,073
SPAGHETTI w/ MUSHROOMS	2.75 OZ.	257	50	18	1	746
PASTA ROMA	3 OZ.	328	47	18	1	686
WHOLE WHEAT PASTA STEW	3 OZ.	275	57	10	1	652
MUSHROOM PILAF W/ VEGETABLES	3.5 OZ.	373	77	41	2	2,196

Table 13-6. Selected Foods and Menus From AlpineAire

Items	Serving Size	Calories per Serving	CHO (grams)	Protein (grams)	Fat (grams)	Sodium (mg)
WILD RICE PILAF W/ALMONDS	3 OZ.	291	89	10	6	1,233
SHRIMP NEWBURG	3 OZ.	318	49	16	6	538
SHRIMP ALFREDO	2.75 OZ.	300	44	18	3	641
TUNA & NOODLES W/CHEESE	2.75 OZ.	325	39	23	7	1,129
CHICKEN ROTELLE	3 OZ.	311	63	25	3	875
SIERRA CHICKEN	3 OZ.	297	50	18	2	671
ALMOND CHICKEN	3.5 OZ.	395	59	21	7	930
CHICKEN PRIMAVERA	2.5 OZ.	266	43	17	2	924
BROWN RICE & CHICKEN W/ VEGETABLES	3.25 OZ.	318	52	17	4	1,230
WILD TYME TURKEY	3.25 OZ.	346	51	18	6	864
MASHED POTA-TOES & GRAVY W/ TURKEY	2.8 OZ.	284	54	11	1	745
TERIYAKI TURKEY	2.75 OZ.	279	46	16	2	929
BEEF STROGA-NOFF W/NOODLES	2.75 OZ.	306	45	22	6	858
COUNTRY BEAN & BEEF CASSEROLE	3 OZ.	282	40	24	4	1,184
BEEF ROTINI	2.75 OZ.	357	58	21	5	466
SIDE DISHES						
VEGETABLE MIX	0.75 OZ.	71	16	3	0.4	65
GARDEN VEGETABLES	0.75 OZ.	79	17	4	0.5	20

Table 13-6. Selected Foods and Menus From AlpineAire

Items	Serving Size	Calories per Serving	CHO (grams)	Protein (grams)	Fat (grams)	Sodium (mg)
POTATOES & CHEDDAR W/ CHIVES	2 OZ.	232	35	8	7	207
PEAS	0.75 OZ.	81	14	6	0.4	2
SWEET CORN	0.75 OZ.	85	20	3	1	
PINTO BEANS	1.25 OZ.	97	18	6	0.4	3
BROCCOLI	0.25 OZ.	25	5	3	0.2	12
CARROTS	0.8 OZ.	71	17	2	0.3	58
WILD RICE	1 OZ.	106	22	4	0.3	1
BROWN RICE	1 OZ.	77	17	2	0.4	0.5
MASHED POTA-TOES	1.75 OZ.	181	42	3.5	0.3	5.25
DICED TURKEY	0.5 OZ.	80	--	13	1	--
DICED CHICKEN	0.5 OZ.	80	--	13	1	--
DICED BEEF	0.5 OZ.	106	--	15	5	30
TOMATO DICES	2 OZ.	43	10	2	1	18
MUSHROOMS	0.5 OZ.	28	4	3	--	15
SWEET BELL PEPPER COMBO	1 OZ.	45	55	2	0.5	23
ONIONS	1.5 OZ.	74	17	2	--	19
TOMATO POWDER	2 OZ.	104	22	5	1	14
CHEDDAR CHEESE POWDER	2 OZ.	164	1	11	14	397
SOUPS						
ALPINE MINESTRONE	1.75 OZ.	159	33	7	2	629
MULTI BEAN SOUP	1.75 OZ.	140	27	9	0.5	823

Table 13-6. Selected Foods and Menus From AlpineAire

Items	Serving Size	Calories per Serving	CHO (grams)	Protein (grams)	Fat (grams)	Sodium (mg)
CREAMY POTATO CHEDDAR SOUP	2 OZ.	225	33	9	7	864
CREAM OF BROCCOLI SOUP	1.25 OZ.	143	19	6	5	861
BREAKFAST ITEMS						
BLUEBERRY PANCAKES	3.25 OZ.	369	63	6	8	0.2
PURE MAPLE SYRUP GRANULES	1.25 OZ.	95	24	--	--	1
RANCH OMELET W/BEEF	2.25 OZ.	399	12	2	25	542
SCRAMBLING & OMELET EGGS	2 OZ.	308	10	20	21	433
BLUEBERRY HONEY GRANOLA & MILK	3.25 OZ.	367	54	15	11	2
STRAWBERRY HONEY GRANOLA & MILK	3.25 OZ.	367	54	15	11	2
FRUITS AND DESSERTS						
APPLE ALMOND CRISP	2.5 OZ.	275	44	6	10	2
APPLESAUCE W/ CINNAMON	1.25 OZ.	125	33	0.5	0.8	3
REAL APPLE-BLUEBERRY FRUIT COBBLER	2 OZ.	210	46	2	2	2
STRAWBERRIES	0.5 OZ.	55	--	1	0.6	30
BLUEBERRIES	0.5 OZ.	60	15	0.7	0.5	1

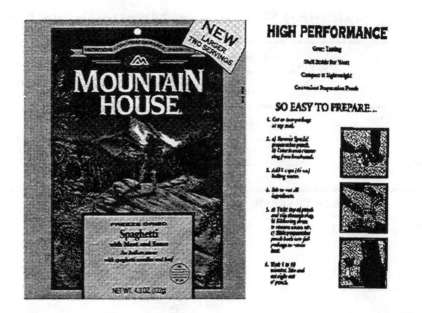

Table 13-7. Selected Foods and Menus From Mountain House

Items	Serving Size (dry wt)	Calories per Serving	CHO (grams)	Protein (grams)	Fat (grams)	Sodium (mg)
BREAKFAST ENTREES						
PRECOOKED EGGS W/BACON	1.3 OZ.	190	6	12	13	920
GRANOLA W/ BLUEBERRIES & MILK	2.0 OZ.	270	38	8	10	60
CHEESE OMELETTE	1.2 OZ.	180	8	13	9	600
EGGS W/BACON	1.1 OZ.	160	6	10	11	750
HASH BROWN POTATOES	2.5 OZ.	150	36	2	0	80
BEEF SAUSAGE PATTIES	0.55 OZ.	80	0	8	5	250

Table 13-7. Selected Foods and Menus From Mountain House

Items	Serving Size (dry wt)	Calories per Serving	CHO (grams)	Protein (grams)	Fat (grams)	Sodium (mg)
VEGETABLES						
CORN	0.75 OZ.	90	18	2	1	1
GREEN PEAS	0.55 OZ.	70	12	4	1	90
GREEN BEANS	0.21 OZ.	35	6	1	0	1
FRUIT & SNACKS						
NUT CHOCOLATE LURPS	1.5 OZ.	250	18	6	17	75
FRUIT CRISPS - STRAWBERRIES	0.5 OZ.	60	13	1	1	0
FRUIT CRISPS - PEACHES	0.55 OZ.	60	15	0	0	5
FRUIT CRISPS - MIXED FRUIT	0.55 OZ.	60	15	0	0	5
FRUIT CRISPS - PEARS	0.5 OZ.	60	14	0	0	0
MAIN COURSE ENTREES						
CHICKEN POLYNESIAN	1.75 OZ.	210	33	10	4	810
GREEN PEPPER & ONION SAUCE W/ BEEF & RICE	1.9 OZ.	230	32	10	7	1200
LASAGNA W/ MEAT & SAUCE	1.8 OZ.	240	23	14	10	630
CHILI MAC W/ BEEF	1.8 OZ.	220	30	12	6	540
BEEF STROGANOFF	1.8 OZ.	250	27	9	12	750
BEEF BOURGUIGNON	2.0 OZ.	280	20	20	13	880
BEEF STEW	1.68 OZ.	260	26	16	9	820

Table 13-7. Selected Foods and Menus From Mountain House

Items	Serving Size (dry wt)	Calories per Serving	CHO (grams)	Protein (grams)	Fat (grams)	Sodium (mg)
SPAGHETTI W/ MEAT & SAUCE	1.7 OZ.	220	27	10	8	940
CHICKEN STEW	1.8 OZ.	230	30	9	8	1200
TURKEY TETRAZINI	1.6 OZ.	210	21	13	8	1150
CHICKEN A LA KING	2.38 OZ.	300	33	18	10	1350
SWEET & SOUR PORK W/RICE	2.3 OZ.	270	44	12	6	730
VEGETABLE STEW W/BEEF	1.7 OZ.	230	27	11	7	580
BEEF & RICE W/ ONIONS	2.4 OZ.	330	42	11	12	1300
RICE & CHICKEN	2.4 OZ.	400	41	13	13	1170
CHILI W/BEANS	2.3 OZ.	310	30	16	14	950
NOODLES & CHICKEN	1.75 OZ.	200	28	13	4	970

What Do You Choose?

The next question you should ask is: Given this information, which is the best product for me to eat during a particular mission scenario? What foods will most impact my performance? The best way to answer that question is to figure out what your expected caloric expenditure will be and what kinds of foods you like! The ration for any mission that involves high activity should provide at least 400 grams of CHO.

Look over some of the food selections provided. What is important is that you eat and drink. Compare the military and commercial foods, and try setting up a menu plan that fits both your personal tastes and energy requirements. The military RCW caloric distribution is a good model to follow, and is an acceptable alternative to store-bought lightweight foods. The Table below provides sample menus for two days; each menu supplies about 4,500 kcal. Use these menus as a template. Other food choices in the preceding tables can be substituted accordingly. There are many types of soups, breakfast products, and dinner entrees to chose from.   The important points to remember are:

◆   Get enough CHO

◆   Drink lots of fluid (preferably low caffeine)

◆   Limit sodium and caffeine intake

Table 13-8. Two Sample Daily Menus for High Activity

DAY 1	DAY 2
Breakfasts - ~1500 kcal, 250 - 270 grams of CHO	
Oatmeal, 3 pkg	Cream of Wheat, 3 pkg
Raisins, 1/2 cup	Honey, 2 Tbsp
Cashews, 1/2 cup	Ranch Omelet w/ Beef, 2.5 oz.
Honey, 2 Tbsp	Applesauce w/ Cinnamon, 1.25 oz.
Cocoa, 2 cup	Cocoa, 2 cups
Orange Drink, 1 cup	Grapefruit Drink, 2 cups
Lunches - ~1600 kcal, 235 - 250 grams of CHO	
Power Bar, 2.25 oz.	Granola Bars, 1 pkg
Raisins, 1/2 cup	Fig Newtons, 6 each
Peanuts, 1/2 cup	Creamy Potato Cheddar Soup, 2.5 oz.
Minestrone Soup, 3.5 oz.	Beef Jerky, 4 oz.
Exceed/Glucose Polymer Beverage, 1 quart	
Dinners - ~1500 kcal, 300 grams of CHO	
Chicken Primavera, 5 oz.	Spaghetti with Mushrooms, 11 oz.
Garden Veggies, 1.5 oz.	Triscuit, 10 each
Apple Almond Crisp 2.5 oz.	Apple/Blueberry Cobbler, 4 oz.
Apple Cider, 2 cups	Apple Cider, 2 cups
Fig Newtons, 6 each	Granola Bars, 1 pkg

An advantage to the military rations is that you don't have to count calories on labels to get the desired caloric distribution. For example: If you are training in a cold weather environment, you know that the RCW has 4,500 kcal/day with an appropriate distribution of calories. There's no need to look at labels three times a day to figure out what you are eating. The time saved by not counting calories may or may not be important to you. However, if you don't like military rations, spend some time developing a meal plan that suits your taste buds, as indicated above. You need to eat on your missions!

Other Ration Information

How Long Will Rations Keep?

As long as the package is left unopened, stored properly in a fairly cool environment (low humidity and less than 80° F), and not handled excessively, most of the military rations will be usable for at least 3 years. The MRE, RLW-30, and RCW all have shelf lives of 3 years. Most commercial foods have expiration dates noted on the packaging, but generally they will also keep for at least 3 years. Mountain House promotes a shelf life of up to 5 years. The ration with the longest shelf life is the improved Long Range Patrol (LRP[I]), which has an estimated life of 10 years at 70 to 80° F.

Rations and Water Requirements

If the rations are prepared as instructed, and you drink fluids as recommended, freeze-dried rations will not increase your need for water. However, if the rations you select contain greater amounts of sodium or protein, you may need additional water.

Chapter 14
Nutritional Considerations For Adverse Conditions

Adverse conditions such as exposure to extreme environments impose considerable physiological demands. The human body responds to adverse conditions by increasing energy expenditure and water losses. If energy and fluid balance is not regained, then performance and perhaps mission integrity can be at stake. In this chapter, information on nutritional interventions that may improve performance or alternatively reduce performance decrements under adverse conditions is presented.

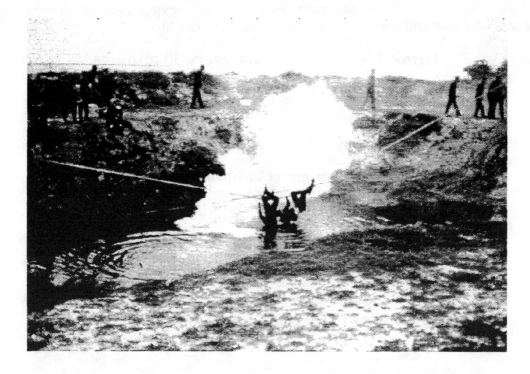

Heat Exposure

Clearly, the major concerns during operations in a warm or hot environment are maintaining fluid and electrolyte balance. Any time you have to work or exercise in the heat, you will lose water and electrolytes through sweating. The amount of sweat produced depends on:

◆ Environmental temperature and humidity

◆ Work rate

◆ Fitness level and acclimatization

◆ Volume and rate of fluid replacement

Working at a high work rate in hot, humid surroundings results in the very high fluid and electrolyte losses. You can easily lose one to two quarts per hour and even more when special clothing, such as chemical protective gear, is required. The highest sweating rate ever reported was 4 quarts per hour.

Fluid Needs

Failure to replace fluids lost through sweating will result in dehydration and eventually heat injury (see Chapters 6 and 11 for additional information on dehydration). Forced drinking is recommended throughout training in a warm environment since your normal thirst mechanism will not ensure adequate fluid replacement.

Drink 1 to 3 cups of fluid every 30 minutes.

More than 3 cups per 30 minutes is TOO MUCH to absorb.

It is a good idea to get a body weight prior to starting a prolonged training mission in the heat, and weigh yourself as time permits. This will allow you to determine your sweat rate and help ensure adequate hydration in later training and simulated operations. Remember that your water needs may be higher when you wear chemical protective clothing or other gear when you work in the heat.

Drink 10 to 12 quarts of water per day at regular intervals when working in a hot environment.

One pound of water loss equals approximately 2 cups of water or about 0.475 quarts.

It is estimated that a water loss of 2% body weight can impair physical performance and mood, decrease appetite and increase the risk of heat injuries. Below is a sample calculation:

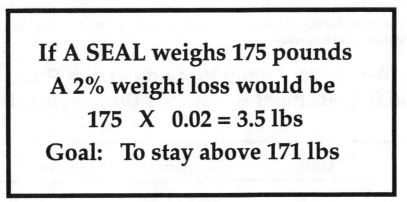

If A SEAL weighs 175 pounds

A 2% weight loss would be

175 X 0.02 = 3.5 lbs

Goal: To stay above 171 lbs

A 5% loss of body weight decreases work performance by 30%. This amount of water loss is a serious threat to your health.

Worksheet 14-1. Calculate Your Lower Weight for Fluid Losses

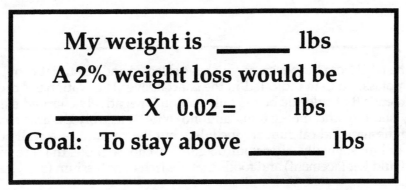

My weight is _____ lbs

A 2% weight loss would be

_____ X 0.02 = _____ lbs

Goal: To stay above _____ lbs

Monitor hydration status by inspecting the color of your urine.

A dark yellow or smelly urine suggests some degree of dehydration; increase fluid consumption until the color becomes pale yellow. If, however, you are taking B vitamins your urine may be not be pale but bright yellow.

Excessive water weight gain can also be a threat to your health. This condition results when individuals drink large amounts of plain water to replace fluid losses during long duration (lasting for 8 or more hours) endurance activities. To prevent overhydration, make sure that you drink beverages that contain electrolytes (sodium and potassium) to replace fluids lost during extended missions.

Electrolyte Balance

It is a fact of life that electrolytes are lost in the sweat, and excessive loss of electrolytes (example: sodium, potassium) can lead to muscle cramping or severe medical problems. However, being in excellent physical condition will help minimize electrolyte losses. The best way to maintain electrolyte balance over prolonged exposure to heat is to drink fluid/electrolyte replacement beverages.

Table 14-1. Upper Limits for Sodium and Potassium in Fluid Replacement Beverages During Heat Stress

Units	Sodium	Potassium
mg/8 oz.	165	46
mg/L	690	195
mEq/8 oz.	7.2	1.2

Look at the label from the beverage you have selected and be sure it provides no more sodium and potassium than indicated in the chart above. The National Academy of Sciences recommends that chloride be the only "anion" (negatively charged electrolyte) accompanying sodium and potassium, and no other electrolytes are recommended. Typically magnesium and calcium are included, but the amounts are well below recommended upper limits. Finally, after your operations, choose foods that are high in water (Chapter 6 - Fluid Replacement) and foods that are rich in potassium (see Chapter 12 and Appendix 6).

Carbohydrate (CHO) Intake

Fluid replacement beverages with CHO are great during exercises in the heat, but the amount of CHO should be lower than usual so that the fluid/water is rapidly absorbed. Chapter 6 provides a chart showing the concentration of CHO in the beverage to use for maintaining hydration status.

> Beverages consumed in the heat should
> be no more than 8% CHO - 5% CHO is optimal

Energy Intake

Although appetites may be suppressed in the hot weather, especially during the first few days after arriving, adequate caloric intake is very important. Inadequate food intake will lead to weight loss which can impair both physical and mental performance. Remember:

Dehydration can result in a loss of appetite.

When you do the same task in a hot environment, energy requirements are slightly increased due to the increased work of maintaining thermal balance. When living/working in temperatures ranging from 86 to 104° F (30 to 40° C) caloric intakes should be increased by 10% as shown below, unless activity level decreases accordingly.

> ## If a SEAL requires 4000 kcal/day
> ## A 10% increase in energy would be
> ## 4000 X 0.10 = 400 kcal/day
> ## Goal: Eat 4400 kcal/day

Worksheet 14-2. Calculate Your Energy Requirements for a Hot Environment

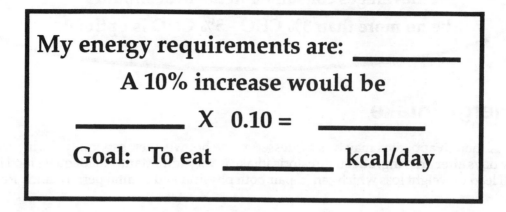

My energy requirements are: _____

A 10% increase would be

_____ X 0.10 = _____

Goal: To eat _____ kcal/day

TIP: If your activity level decreases you do not need any extra calories.

Other Recommendations:

◆ Eat a high CHO diet as they are absorbed more readily than fat and protein.

◆ Avoid fatty foods which may not be not well tolerated in the heat.

◆ Avoid high or excessive protein intakes which will increase water loss and can lead to dehydration.

Cold Exposure

Exposure to a cold environment, be it air or water, is a challenge to be taken very seriously; performance decrements are common when you become cold. The body's response to cold exposure is a "tightening of blood vessels" to conserve heat, and shivering to generate heat and guard against hypothermia (a dangerously low core body temperature). Side effects of these responses are an increased in urine output and an increase in energy metabolism. Therefore, the most important aspects of nutrition in a cold environment are:

◆ Energy intake

◆ Fluid status

◆ Vitamin and mineral needs

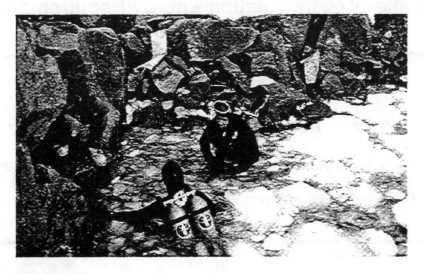

Energy Intake

Energy requirements can increase 25 to 50% during cold weather operations as compared to warm weather operations.

A 3 to 4° decrease in body temperature can result in a two to fourfold increase in resting energy expenditure. That's a huge increase in the body's metabolic rate. Factors that increase calorie needs include:

◆ Added exertion due to wearing heavy gear

◆ Shivering which can increase resting metabolic rate by two to four times above normal

◆ Increased activity associated with traveling over snow and icy terrain

◆ Increased activity to keep warm

Many studies have shown that soldiers tend to progressively lose weight when conducting field exercises in the cold for 2 to 3 weeks. Because significant weight loss can result in fatigue and performance decrements, energy intake must increase to meet the increased energy demands.

Both fats and CHO are used as fuel when exposed to a cold environment. However, a high CHO diet is preferred as it will replenish glycogen stores that are rapidly being used to maintain core temperature. A high fat diet is discouraged as it would require a prolonged period of adaptation and may result in gastrointestinal problems. Ideally 60% of your energy should come from CHO, 30% from fat and 10% from protein, with high CHO snacks eaten in between meals. Protein supplements or high protein diets are not recommended as they would increase water losses.

Table 14-2. Calculating Energy Requirements for Cold Weather

If a SEAL requires 4000 kcal/day

A 25% increase in energy would be

4000 X 0.25 = 1000 kcal

Goal: Eat 4000 + 1000 or 5000 kcal/day

Eat frequent snacks during the day and a large snack before going to bed

Fluid Status

Becoming dehydrated in cold environments is very easy because of the cold-induced increase in urine output, increased fluid losses through breathing, involuntary reduction in fluid intake, and sweating. Because dehydration will decrease performance and potentially lead to various medical problems, maintenance of fluid status by drinking plenty of fluids and monitoring hydration status is absolutely critical (see Chapter 6).

Tips for Maintaining Fluid Status

◆ Force yourself to drink 2 to 4 cups of warm fluid at hourly intervals.

◆ Avoid alcoholic beverages as alcohol tends to increase heat and urine losses.

◆ Moderate caffeine consumption since caffeine increases fluid losses.

◆ Avoid consuming salty foods that increase fluid needs.

◆ Drink beverages with CHO to increase energy intake.

◆ Don't eat snow without first melting and purifying it.

Vitamin and Mineral Needs

When working in the cold, the requirements for some vitamins and minerals may increase to meet the demands of increased energy metabolism (example: thiamin) or greater urinary losses (example: magnesium, zinc). The amount by which daily vitamin and mineral needs may increase above the RDA (see Chapter 3 for RDAs) during cold weather operations was recently proposed: suggested amounts are shown in the Table below. These amounts are based on intake data from field studies, urinary excretion of nutrients and other measures of "nutrient status". In most cases, if you meet your energy requirements by eating all ration components you should be able to meet your vitamin and mineral needs.

Table 14-3. Suggested Increases in Daily Intakes of Vitamins and Minerals During Cold Exposure

Nutrient	Suggested Increase	% of RDA
Vitamin B_1 (Thiamin)	3 mg	200
Vitamin B_2 (Riboflavin)	2 mg	118
Vitamin B_3	5 mg	26
Pantothenic Acid	5 mg	100
Folic Acid	200 µg	100
Vitamin B_{12}	1 µg	50
Magnesium	200 mg	57
Zinc	5 mg	33

Sustained Operations

Sustained Operations (SUSOPS) are work periods of 12 hours or more that usually result in physical and mental fatigue and sleep loss. In contrast, Continuous Operations (CONOPS) are periods of uninterrupted activity of "normal shift length" followed by sufficient sleep. Your missions, which usually include both SUSOPS and CONOPS, frequently result in fatigue and sleep loss. Nutritional interventions can partially offset the effects of fatigue and sleep deprivation on physical and mental performance. The most effective nutritional interventions include:

◆ CHO intake

◆ Hydration status

◆ Caffeine intake

CHO Intake

A high CHO diet is needed for replacing muscle glycogen stores that are used up during prolonged activity and for maintaining a sufficient "blood glucose" level. Thus, your diet during SUSOPS should provide 60 to 65% of energy from CHO, 10% from protein and the remaining calories from fat.

High CHO snacks or CHO-containing fluid replacement beverages providing 15 to 30 g of CHO/hour will also help to maintain blood glucose and delay fatigue during strenuous prolonged missions (see Chapters 6 and 9 for additional information). When blood glucose levels fall, your performance will drop rapidly, and you will become unable to continue working.

Table 14-4. Symptoms of Hypoglycemia
(low blood sugar)

Headache	**Blurred vision**
Weakness	**Confusion**
Dizziness	**Unconsciousness**
Fatigue	**Sweating**

CHO loading can be useful when preparing for missions that require continuous movement such as snow shoeing, skiing, swimming, trekking over difficult terrain etc. for a few hours in order to reach the objective (see Chapter 9 for information on CHO loading).

Nutritional Considerations For Adverse Conditions

Caffeine

If you are a regular user of caffeine, it will not do much to "pick you up" but if you discontinue caffeine use, it may cause discomfort. In general, caffeine increases urine output and could cause dehydration. However, you may want to try some caffeine to see if it increases your alertness and delays fatigue during extended operations. See Chapter 15 for the caffeine content of various beverages and medications.

Fluid Intake

On some training and actual missions water may not be available. Thus, prior hydration will assume a greater importance. When water or beverages are available it is important to remain well hydrated given that dehydration can decrease both mental and physical performance (see Chapter 6).

Forced drinking of 1 to 3 cups per 30 minutes, depending on the temperature, is recommended.

Beverages containing 5 to 8% CHO and some electrolytes are best.

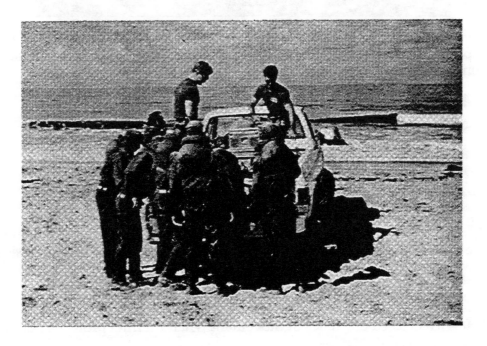

Diving and Immersion in Water

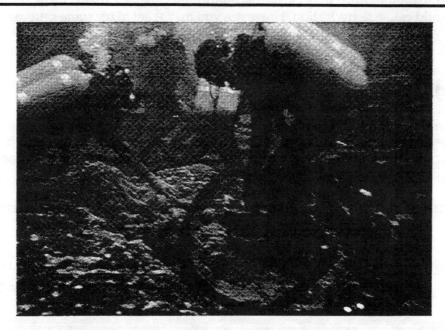

Like exposure to altitude and a cold environment, water operations, especially cold water operations, are associated with increased energy expenditure and fluid losses. Thus nutritional concerns for diving are maintenance of:

♦ Energy intake

♦ Fluid intake

♦ Replacing mineral losses

Energy Intake

When working at the same rate in water as on land, the energy expenditure to accomplish the same task is greater in water. The reasons for this increased energy expenditure during water operations include:

♦ Greater resistance offered by water

♦ Decreased efficiency of movement when thermal protective clothing are worn

This is especially true in cold water. To meet the increased energy requirements you may need to increase your intake of CHO. If the water is cold, this is very important.

Tips for maintaining performance in cold water

◆ Eat a high CHO diet (see Chapters 2, 9 and 11).

◆ Consider CHO loading for extended dives

Glycogen stores are rapidly used when performing hard work in cold water. These stores must be replaced between operations to prevent performance decrements (see Chapter 9). CHO loading before an anticipated dive has been shown to improve and extend exercise performance during prolonged dives and has been discussed in Chapter 9.

Fluid Intake

Immersion in water increases urinary output by 2 to 10 times above normal. Without adequate hydration a diver can quickly become dehydrated and suffer performance decrements. For example, immersion during a single dive for 3 to 6 hours can result in a 2 to 8 pound loss in body weight by urination; this is equivalent to losing 1 to 3 quarts of fluid.

Although fluid ingestion during immersion has not been found to improve hydration status during short term dives (less than 3 hours), attempts to drink fluids with CHO should proceed whenever possible to maintain blood glucose. A decline in blood glucose is known to adversely affect performance.

Mineral Needs

Immersion in water, especially in cold water, can increase urinary losses of magnesium, calcium, zinc and chromium; see Chapter 3 and Appendix 6 for good food sources and recommended intakes.

Altitude

Ascent to altitude can cause a variety of disturbances, and adequate nutrition can play a crucial role in maintaining performance. The major nutritional concerns at altitude are:

◆ Weight loss

◆ CHO intake

◆ Dehydration

◆ Disturbances in digestion

◆ Vitamin and mineral needs

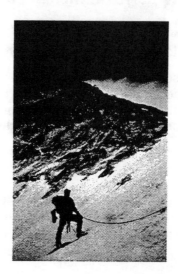

Weight Loss

Virtually all persons who go to altitude experience weight loss and loss of lean body mass. At altitudes below 5000 m weight loss can be prevented by increased caloric intake, whereas above 5000 m, a 5 to 10% weight loss is almost inevitable. Some reasons for weight loss at high-altitude are:

◆ Energy requirements are increased 15 to 50% above sea level

◆ Decreased sense of taste causing a reduction in food intake

◆ Loss of body water from increased breathing rate and dry air

◆ Impaired absorption of nutrients

◆ Acute Mountain Sickness (AMS) which can result in nausea, vomiting, headache and decreased appetite

The only way to minimize weight loss is by increasing your energy intake.

Energy requirements can increase 15 to 50% above requirements at sea level.

Recommended caloric intakes range from 3500 to 6000 calories per day; this is equivalent to eating at least four MREs or one Ration,Cold Weather daily.

Table 14-5. Calculating Energy Requirements at Altitude

> **If a SEAL requires 3000 kcal/day**
>
> **A 50% increase in energy would be**
>
> **3000 X   0.50 = 1500 kcal**
>
> **Goal: Eat 4500 kcal/day**

Tips for Maintaining Energy Balance

◆ Eat small frequent meals.

◆ Protein should constitute no more than 10% of the daily caloric intake. Higher intakes will be excreted along with water.

◆ Fatty foods may not be well tolerated at altitude and may exaccerbate AMS.

CHO Intake

High CHO foods are the preferred energy source at altitude because they:

◆ Replete glycogen stores - glycogen stores are depleted in a couple of hours by strenuous physical activity

◆ Require less oxygen (which is decreased at altitude) than fat to burn and are therefore, the more efficient energy source.

◆ Can blunt and delay the progression or severity of symptoms of AMS (nausea, vomiting, headache).

You should derive 60% of calories or at least 400 g from CHO diet. This can be accomplished by eating high CHO snacks (see Chapter 7) between meals and drinking CHO-containing beverages during strenuous activity and recovery (see Chapter 6 for recommended rehydration practices).

Dehydration

Water losses are increased at altitude and if these losses are not replaced dehydration results. As stated several times before, dehydration impairs physical and mental performance and increases the risk of cold injury. Dehydration occurs at altitude for several reasons:

◆ Increased respiratory losses due to increased ventilation

◆ Increased urine output due to altitude and cold temperatures

◆ Possible diarrheal fluid losses

◆ Failure to drink water

◆ Meeting the increased fluid needs can be a challenge since thirst does not always keep pace with needs

> ## Fluid requirements may be 4.25 quarts or more per day at high altitude

> ## A drinking schedule must be established and hydration status should be monitored daily.

Vitamin and Mineral Needs

As discussed in the section on cold, vitamin and mineral needs are likely to be increased at altitude where it is cold and oxygen availability is decreased. In particular, increased metabolic rate and hypoxic conditions at altitude can increase the production of harmful free radicals which may slow blood circulation and impair physical performance. Preliminary findings indicate that taking vitamin E (400 IU/day) at high altitude reduces free radical production, and helps maintain blood flow and aerobic energy metabolism in men.

Summary

Energy and fluid requirements are higher than normal during all the scenarios described in this chapter (see each section for estimated increases). Importantly, weight loss due to inadequate energy intake and/or dehydration can result in fatigue and impaired performance. Therefore, keys to being nutritionally prepared during training and missions in adverse environments are:

◆ Meet energy needs preferably by **eating a high CHO diet**. Eat high CHO snacks to meet increased energy needs.

◆ **Be well hydrated** - Follow a forced fluid replacement schedule since thirst is not a good indicator of fluid needs.

◆ Avoid protein supplements as the extra protein is excreted along with water and can be dehydrating.

Chapter 15
Ergogenic Agents - Looking for "The Edge"

*E*rgogenic agents are by definition, substances or techniques that enhance performance. Because SEALs are required to perform at a high level both mentally and physically, many are looking for substances or techniques to improve performance and provide "an edge". To perform longer, to be faster, to be stronger, and to be leaner, if not a mission goal, are personal goals of many SEALs and elite athletes. People have been trying to accomplish these goals for centuries through the use of ergogenic agents. It is the goal of this chapter to present information and comments about certain products commonly found in retail stores or by mail order, that claim performance enhancing effects.

The comments in this chapter are based on the most up-to-date objective scientific information, although in some cases limited information is available, and most have not been tested for their ability to enhance SEAL or Special Operations mission-related performance. Some products are unlikely to hurt you, and you will have to decide if you want to try it, whereas other products may be harmful and you may be strongly discouraged from trying it. In many cases you may be using supplements that are a waste of money. This chapter will assist you in making good decisions.

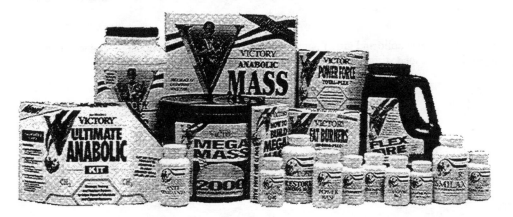

Nutritional Products Advertised as Ergogenic Agents

This section lists many of the nutritional ergogenic agents sold by manufacturers with claims to "enhance performance" or have "muscle building" properties. Some have valid claims whereas others do not. It is often difficult to differentiate false claims from valid ones if you haven't carefully researched each product individually. Many claims sound very scientific and convincing but, unfortunately, they are often false or unproven. For each agent described below, the claims, the usual dose used, and a comment are provided. Remember, if the comment is NO, the product may be harmful.

Table 15-1. Nutritional Ergogenic Agents

AGENTS	CLAIMS	DOSE	COMMENT
Arginine, Lysine, and Ornithine	Stimulate growth hormone release.	Variable. Arginine - 500 mg. one hour before meals and/or before workout. Ornithine - 500 mg. a day or 250 mg. one to three times a day. These items are sold separately or in combinations with varying amounts of amino acid content.	Ornithine - No. Gastro-intestinal disturbances are common. Arginine, Lysine - Some benefit reported.
Sodium Bicarbonate, ("Bicarb loading", "Soda loading")	Enhances anaerobic performance during high intensity exercise lasting 1 to 5 minutes.	0.3 grams of Sodium Bicarb per kg body weight mixed with 1 liter of water 1 to 2 hours before exercise.	Some benefit reported - Be careful...harmful if taken in large amounts. Discontinue use if abdominal cramps or diarrhea occurs.
Branched Chain Amino Acids (BCAAs) - Leucine, Isoleucine, Valine	Anabolic and growth hormone stimulator; may protect against mental fatigue of exercise.	There are various products with different amounts of BCAA in them. Here's an example: Leucine 800 mg. daily. Isoleucine 300 mg. Valine 200 mg. These are usually consumed prior to working out. Foods rich in BCAAs include turkey, chicken, navy beans, and other meats.	Some benefits reported.

Table 15-1. Nutritional Ergogenic Agents

AGENTS	CLAIMS	DOSE	COMMENT
Caffeine	Delays fatigue, enhances performance, "burns" fat.	4 to 9 mg/kg 30 minutes to one hour prior to exercise. Look at the caffeine levels in some common beverages.	Some benefits reported, but discontinue use if side effects (stomach pain, tremor) interfere with concentration or steadiness.
L-Carnitine	"Fat burner", delays onset of fatigue.	500 mg daily. Foods rich in Carnitine include beef (average content equals 50 mg/100 grams of edible portion).	Little to no benefit reported - not harmful at recommended doses. AVOID D-carnitine - a carnitine deficiency may occur.
Choline	Enhances endurance performance	400 to 900 mg daily as choline bitartrate. Foods rich in choline include meat, liver, and peanuts.	No benefit reported - not known to be harmful at above doses. Most claims based on theoretical possibilities.
Chromium Picolinate	Increases muscle mass, growth stimulating.	50 to 1000 µg/day as a dietary supplement. Foods rich in chromium include beer, brewer's yeast, oysters, mushrooms, meats, and whole grain cereals.	Some benefit reported.
Coenzyme Q10	Increases energy and cardiac performance. Potent antioxidant.	1.0 mg three times a day. Foods rich in CoQ10 include beef, eggs, and spinach.	No benefit reported in athletes.
Dibencozide or cobamamide - Coenzyme forms of B_{12}	Anabolic and growth promoting.	500 mg daily in tablet form.	Little or no proven benefit - no harmful effects at recommended doses.
λ–Oryzanol and Ferulic Acid	Increases testosterone and increases lean body mass.	Variable, but commonly found in 50 mg per day doses.	Little or no proven benefit - no harmful effects at given doses.

Table 15-1. Nutritional Ergogenic Agents

AGENTS	CLAIMS	DOSE	COMMENT
Glandulars (ground up animal organs usually testes, pituitary, or hypothalamus)	Will elevate your testosterone levels. This "extra" testosterone will make you more anabolic (build up) and get bigger.	As a dietary supplement mixed with protein/carbohydrate powders.	Truly not worth the money!
Inosine	Energy enhancer; Increases endurance, strength, and recuperation.	500 to 1000 mg 15 minutes prior to exercise.	No. People with gout should avoid inosine. Dubious effects not worth the risk.
Octacosanol - Wheat Germ Oil	Improves endurance capacity.	100 to 6000 mg daily with expected results in 4 to 6 weeks.	Some benefit reported.
Sapogenins - Smilax, Diascorea, Trillium, Yucca, or Sarsaparilla	Increases muscle mass and lean body weight by increasing testosterone levels. A testosterone precursor.	Sublingual or capsular as directed. Use prior to workout and before bed.	Little benefit reported. Some products suspended in 18% alcohol. READ the label.
Tyrosine	Reverses cold induced working memory deficit. Positive impact on stress induced cognitive performance degradation.	75 to 150 mg/kg of L-tyrosine 1 to 2 hours prior to exposure.	Some benefits reported in SEAL cold weather operations. Branch chained amino acids should not be taken with tyrosine since they will interfere with tyrosine's action.

Table 15-2. Caffeine Content of Selected Beverages, Products, and Medications

Coffee (8 oz.)	mg	Soda (12 oz.)*	mg
Percolated	102 - 200	Mountain Dew	55
Drip	176 - 240	Coke	46
Instant	64 - 176	Dr. Pepper	40
Decaffeinated	3.2 - 8	Pepsi	38
Tea (8 oz.)		Mellow Yellow	52
3-Minute Brew	32 - 74	Mr. Pibb	50
Instant	24 - 45	**Chocolate (1 oz.)**	25
Iced	35 - 58	**Pain Relievers (1 tablet)**	
Stimulants (1 tablet)		Anacin	32
No Doz	100	Excedrin	65
Vivarin	200	Dristan	0

*Sugar-free and diet versions of above sodas have same caffeine content as original.

Table 15-3. Summary of Ergogenic Agents

Agent	Comment
Delays Fatigue/Increases Energy Levels	
Caffeine	Some benefits reported
Choline	No benefit reported
Coenzyme Q_{10}	No proven benefit
Inosine	No proven benefit
Octacosanol	Some benefit reported

Agent	Comment
Sodium Bicarbonate	Some reported benefit
Tyrosine	Some benefits reported during SEAL cold weather ops

Fat Burners/Lean Body Mass Increasers

Carnitine	Little or no benefit reported
Chromium	Some benefit reported
λ-Oryzanol/Ferulic Acid	Little or no benefit reported

Testosterone Enhancers

Glandulars	Not recommended
Hot Stuff	Possible adverse effects
Smilax	Little or no benefit reported

Growth Hormone Releasers

Arginine	Some benefit reported
Branch Chain Amino Acids	Some benefit reported
Dibencozide	Little or no proven benefit
Lysine	Some benefit reported

Protein- Carbohydrate Supplements

Go into a retail or specialty store that caters to athletes and you may become overwhelmed by the number of different products available. One of the most highly visible and advertised group of products are the powdered protein and carbohydrate beverages. "Weight gaining", "anabolic", "muscle building"- these are just a few of the various claims made by manufacturers. They do share one thing in common however: they are sold as supplements to your diet. These products are intended to fortify your diet to meet the nutrient demands of your body. In general, there are three basic reasons why people supplement:

◆ Compensate for less than adequate diets or life-styles

◆ Meet unusual nutrient demands induced by heavy exercise and/or

◆ Produce direct positive effects on performance.

Your profession and life-style impose unique physical demands that require stamina, power, and strength. Consequently, your caloric (energy) expenditure is greater than the average person.

In Chapter 1 you calculated your REE and then, based on your activity level, your total daily caloric expenditure. Do you think your caloric intake supports your activity level? If not, you have two methods to increase your energy intake:

◆ You can eat more (which can be difficult based on your daily schedule)

◆ You can use a supplement to make up for the extra calories you need.

Supplements are a quick and convenient means for obtaining the nutrients you need. For example, some people find that after eating a normal breakfast they feel ill or nauseous during morning PT. If you can't tolerate exercising on a full stomach, then a powdered beverage may be the answer for your breakfast. You get the calories you need in the morning, but don't have that heavy feeling in your stomach. Remember that you may not need the full recommended serving size. Count the calories to suit your own energy requirements and goals.

It is also important to realize that it is not the supplement alone that leads to better performance. Success lies in addressing your goals and analyzing and adapting your diet to meet those goals. It will take some work on your part to calculate how much supplement, if any, you need to use. Read the labels and figure out how many calories you will expend before your next meal. Also, make sure you add up the vitamins and minerals you are getting from all the different supplements you are taking. Many products provide similar nutrients and you may be taking TOO much of one or several nutrients.

Another decision to make is whether or not to use a protein, carbohydrate, or combination beverage. Once again, it all depends on your goals. If you want to increase lean body mass through resistive training, then some protein may be the way to go. Remember:

All you need is 0.6 to 0.8 grams of protein per pound body weight per day

If you need more than you can eat, then a supplement with protein may be for you. Many powders contain both protein and carbohydrate in a good ratio. Find the one that has the most appropriate amount of each to augment your diet (Refer to Chapter 10 for a list of Protein and Carbohydrate Supplements).

Here is an example: The goal of a 24 year old SEAL who weighs 175 lbs, is to increase his lean body mass through weight training. He knows that he needs between 0.6 and 0.8 and NO MORE than 1.0 grams of protein per pound to achieve this goal. He decides to eat 0.8 grams of protein per pound to see if he'll achieve his goals. His protein requirements are calculated as shown:

---

175 X 0.8 grams protein = desired protein intake

175 lbs X 0.8 = 140 grams of protein daily.

NO MORE THAN 175 X 1 or 175 grams of protein.

Now let's see how much protein he eats on an average day

Breakfast		Afternoon Snack	
Sausage McMuffin	23 g	2 Sports bars	20 g
10 oz. milk	12 g		
1 bagel	6 g	Dinner	
		1 1/2 Chicken Breast	80 g
Mid morning Snack		Broccoli	3 g
1 Yogurt	8 g	Baked Potato	2 g
Lunch			
Big Mac	25 g	Total Protein Intake	212 g
Cheeseburger	18 g	Calculated Requirements	140 g
Fries	6 g		
Shake	9 g		

MET-Rx

MET-Rx is a nutritional supplement with claims of decreasing body fat and increasing muscle mass, if used in conjunction with a regular exercise program. The exercise program is primarily strength/resistive (weight) training. As with any supplement, it is designed to augment your normal diet to meet the increased nutritional demands of exercise. However, increased nutritional needs can also easily be met by dietary means.

The cornerstone of Met-Rx is that it is a high protein supplement (see nutritional information below). The protein is in the form of egg whites, whey protein concentrate, and Metamyosin™ which is claimed to be a "unique blend of milk protein isolates".

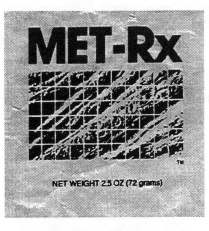

NET WEIGHT 2.5 OZ (72 grams)

Table 15-4. Ingredients in One Serving of MET-Rx

Energy-Providing Nutrients	
Carbohydrates	24 grams
Protein	37 grams
Fat	2 grams
Total Calories	262 kcal
Selected Vitamins and Minerals (% US RDA)	
Vitamin A	40
Vitamin B$_6$	60
Vitamin B$_{12}$	50
Vitamin C	60
Vitamin D	60
Chromium	50 µg

Depending on your goals, MET-Rx may or may not be for you. For example, if you are interested in improving aerobic endurance MET-Rx alone is a poor source of the necessary carbohydrates for that kind of activity. If, however, increasing muscle mass is your goal, then this product provides protein for that. Remember that you don't need more than 0.8 grams of protein per pound body weight.

One major drawback of MET-Rx is the cost. Each serving is roughly $3.00 and the directions for use call for 2 to 4 servings a day. That averages to about $9.00 a day! Keep in mind that there are always alternative sources of protein that are very easy to come by and tend to be much less money. For example,

♦ One can of tuna fish has 36 grams of protein,

♦ One 4 oz. breast of chicken has 36 grams of protein

♦ One 8 oz. glass of milk (skim) has 10 grams of protein.

Remember: There is nothing "magical "about this product and all the ingredients are found in nature. Record your intake and see if it is worth your money.

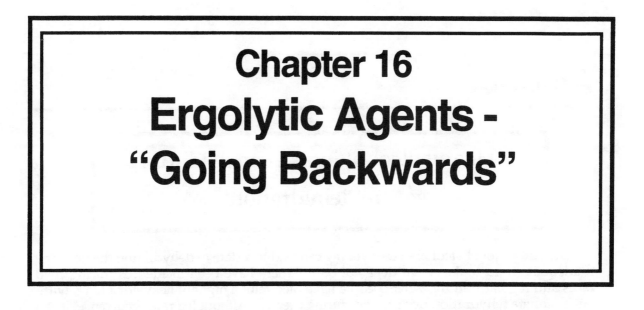

Chapter 16
Ergolytic Agents -
"Going Backwards"

After reading about agents that are potentially beneficial to you, its now time to focus on substances that can destroy what you've been trying to build up. *Ergolytic agents* are those substances which do not enhance, but rather impair, performance, be it physical, mental, or psychological. When using these substances, you may be undoing the benefits and successes gained through training and the use of ergogenic agents. Here's another way to think of it -- you may be wasting your money if on one hand you are buying ergogenic agents and on the other continuing to use ergolytic agents. Hopefully, by staying away from ergolytic agents, you can maximally improve your athletic performance

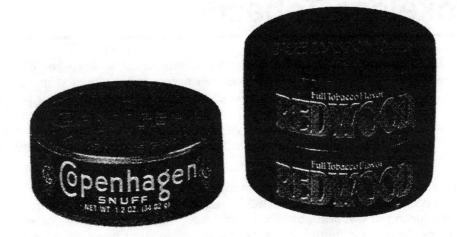

Alcohol

> ## Heavy alcohol intake can lead to severe dehydration!

Drinking a lot of alcohol in the evening can lead to a state of dehydration the next day if adequate fluid replacement does not occur. There have been incidences during road races and regular training where people have died after a night of heavy drinking, without adequate rehydration prior to and during exercise. Although a rare occurrence, it can happen.

Some athlete believe that drinking small amount of alcohol prior to an event can be relaxing and instill self-confidence. *This is completely false.* In fact, alcohol may compromise physical performance by decreasing the release of glucose from the liver. This will cause a decrease in blood glucose and possibly lead to hypoglycemia.

Numerous studies on young trained athletes have shown that performance decreases after ingestion of alcohol. The myth that alcohol can alter the perception of fatigue is also false. There is generally no effect on perception of performance after drinking.

Smokeless Tobacco

Many SEALs have been or are frequent users of smokeless tobacco. Use of such products has been on the rise in the past 20 years with an annual reported increase of 11% since 1974. Many athletes believe that smokeless tobacco will improve their performance or enhance their reaction time by giving them a quick "rush" during the event. After a brief discussion of what nicotine (the active ingredient in all tobacco products) does to your body, you will understand why performance enhancement and chew don't go together.

Nicotine is the major ingredient of smokeless tobacco and very, very addictive (as addicting as cocaine or heroin). It is termed *a psychoactive drug* which means it alters the normal functioning of the brain by stimulating the central nervous system and resulting in the nicotine "buzz" or "high". It is this "mental state" that users claim enhances their reaction time and performance. However, studies have shown no differences in reaction times between users and non-users of smokeless tobacco. Remember: there are NO reaction time improvements with chew.

Nicotine has some very detrimental effects on an athlete. Nicotine is a vasoconstrictor (makes blood vessels tighten). This action on the circulatory system raises blood pressure and heart rate, thereby causing a decrease in cardiac efficiency. In one study of young athletes, two parameters of cardiac performance (stroke volume - the amount of blood pumped out of the heart with each contraction, and cardiac output - the amount of blood the heart pumps in one minute) both showed decreases while using smokeless tobacco. This is very undesirable for an athlete and could cause a severe decrease in performance.

Antihistamines

Antihistamine use is prevalent among all groups of people since it is a common over-the-counter medication. Many types of antihistamines are used, with the most common ones being Benadryl and Seldane. One of the most common side effects of many antihistamines is **drowsiness.** This is not typically seen with many of the newer, "non-sedating" types of antihistamines.

> ## Antihistamines may compromise mental performance

Some of the detrimental mental effects of the sedating antihistamines include:

- ◆ Decreased ability to concentrate
- ◆ Increase in reaction time
- ◆ Sleepiness
- ◆ Decreased score on rifle target practice - "more misses"

Seldane appears to have the least effects in terms of drowsiness and mental performance decrements, so if you need an antihistamine, it may be best to take this one!

Other Side Effects of Sedating Antihistamines

Dry Mouth	Increase in Heart Rate
Blurred Vision	Constipation

No clear cut effects on physical performance have been observed, but caution should be exerted when taking any type of medication.

Appendix 1
Carbohydrate Content of Selected Foods

Food Items[1]	Amount of Food Items (cooked or prepared)	Total Calories	CHO (g)	% Calories from CHO
BEANS/ LENTILS/ DRIED PEAS				
Baked beans, canned	1 cup	236	52.1	78.0
Black beans	1 cup	225	41	72.9
Chickpeas	1 cup	270	45	66.7
Green peas	1 cup	115	21	73.0
Kidney beans	1 cup	230	42	73.0
Lentils	1 cup	215	38	70.7
Lima beans	1 cup	260	49	75.4
Navy beans	1 cup	225	40	71.1
Pinto beans	1 cup	265	49	74.0
Refried beans	1 cup	295	51	69.2
BREADS and GRAINS				
Bagel	1 each	200	38	76.0
Biscuits	1 each	95	14.	58.9
Bread, cracked wheat	1 slice	65	11	67.7

Food Items[1]	Amount of Food Items (cooked or prepared)	Total Calories	CHO (g)	% Calories from CHO
Bread, mixed grain	1 slice	65	11	67.7
Bread, oatmeal	1 slice	65	12	73.8
Bread, raisin	1 slice	65	13	80.0
Bread, whole wheat	1 slice	70	13	74.3
English muffin	1 each	140	27	77.1
Pita bread, white	80.0	165	33	80.0
Pasta, egg noodles	1 cup	200	37	74.0
Spaghetti, enriched	1 cup	155	32	82.6
Rice cake cracker	2 each	70	15.2	86.9
Rice, white	1 cup	225	50	88.9
Rice, brown long grain	1 cup	216	44.8	83.0

CEREALS and BREAKFAST FOODS

Food Items[1]	Amount of Food Items (cooked or prepared)	Total Calories	CHO (g)	% Calories from CHO
All Bran	1 oz	110	21	76.4
40% Bran Flakes	1 oz	102	22	86.2
Cheerios	1 oz	110	20	72.7
Granola, Nature Valley	1 oz	125	19	60.8
Grape-Nuts	1 oz	100	23	92.0
Oatmeal, nonfortified	1 cup	145	25	69.0
Pancakes from mix, no syrup	3 medium	249	33	53
Raisin Bran	1 oz	90	21	74.5
Shredded Wheat	1 biscuit	83	18.8	85.0
Special K	1 oz	110	21	74.5
Total	1 oz	100	22	88.0
Waffles from mix, no syrup	2 large	410	54	52.7
Wheaties	1 oz	100	23	92.0

Food Items[1]	Amount of Food Items (cooked or prepared)	Total Calories	CHO (g)	% Calories from CHO
DAIRY PRODUCTS				
Buttermilk	1 cup	99	11.7	48.6
Cottage Cheese, Regular	l cup	232	6.2	10.7
Cottage Cheese, Low-fat (1%)	1 cup	164	6.2	15.1
Ice cream	1 cup	264	31	47.0
Ice milk	1 cup	184	30	65.2
Milkshake, vanilla	12 oz	380	60.4	63.5
Milk, Whole	l cup	150	11.4	30.4
Milk, 2% Low-fat	1 cup	121	11.7	38.6
Milk, skim nonfat	1 cup	86	11.8	54.9
Milk, regular chocolate	1 cup	208	25.8	49.6
Yogurt, regular, plain	8 oz	139	10.6	30.5
Yogurt, fruit flavored	8 oz	253	42.7	67.5
Yogurt, nonfat plain	8 oz	127	17.4	54.8
FRUITS/VEGETABLES				
Apple, raw	l medium	80	20	100
Avocado	l medium	306	12	15.6
Banana	l medium	127	33.0	94.5
Broccoli, raw	l stalk	32	5.9	75.0
Cantaloupe	1 cup	56	13.3	99
Carrots, raw	1 large	42	9.7	92.3
Cauliflower, raw	1/2 cup	13	2.6	80
Corn, cooked	1 cup	134	33.7	100
Grapefruit	1 medium	78	19.8	90
Grapes, red seedless	1/2 cup	29	7.9	100

Food Items[1]	Amount of Food Items (cooked or prepared)	Total Calories	CHO (g)	% Calories from CHO
Oranges	1 medium	64	16.0	99
Orange juice	1 cup	110	26.1	99
Pear, D'Anjou	1 medium	118	30.1	99
Pineapple juice	1 cup	140	34.5	99
Plum	1 medium	36	8.6	100
Potato, baked	1 large	145	32.8	90.5
Raisins, seedless	1/4 cup	109	28.8	99
Sweet Potato, baked	1 medium	117	27.7	94.7
Tomato juice	1 cup	42	10.3	99
Tomato, raw	1 medium	25	5	80
MISCELLANEOUS				
Angelfood cake	1 slice	129	29.3	90.8
Cheesecake	1 slice	256	20.4	31.8
Doughnuts, plain cake	1 each	198	23.4	47.3
Fig Newtons	2 each	112	22.6	80.7
Popcorn, plain	1 cup	25	5	80
Pretzels, Dutch	2 each	120	24	80

[1]Information for meats, fish and poultry is not provided since the contribution from CHO is typically < 1% of the energy.

Appendix 2
Fat Content of Selected Foods

Food Items[1]	Amount of Food Items (cooked or prepared)	Total Calories	Fats (g)	% Calories from Fat
BEEF				
Hamburger, lean ground beef, broiled	4 oz	307	21.3	62.4
Roast Beef	4 oz	420	34	72.8
Steak, sirloin broiled	4 oz	320	20.4	57.4
LAMB				
Lamb Chop, loin broiled	4 oz	336	16	42.9
Lamb Rib roasted	4 oz	420	34	72.8
PORK				
Bacon, regular	3 strips	110	9	81.8
Bacon, Canadian style	2 slices	85	4	42.4
Bologna	2 slices	180	16	80
Ham, roasted	4 oz	273	13.8	45.4
Hot Dog	1 each	145	13	80.7
Luncheon Meat	2 slices	140	13	83.6

Food Items[1]	Amount of Food Items (cooked or prepared)	Total Calories	Fats (g)	% Calories from Fat
Pork chop, broiled	4 oz	392	30.8	70.7
Salami	2 slices	145	11.9	74.5
POULTRY				
Chicken, breast roasted w/o skin	4 oz	187	4	19.3
Turkey, light meat	4 oz	180	3.7	18.5
Turkey, dark meat	4 oz	213	8.2	34.6
FISH AND SHELLFISH				
Fish Sticks	1 each	70	3.2	40.6
Halibut, broiled	4 oz	187	8	38.5
Oysters, raw	1/2 cup	160	4.4	24.7
Salmon, canned	1 cup	160	6.2	34.9
Sardines, canned	4 oz	233	13.0	50.2
Tuna, water packed	4 oz	180	1.3	6.5
Tuna, oil packed	4 oz	220	9.3	38.0
DAIRY PRODUCTS				
Buttermilk	1 cup	99	2.2	20
Cheese, American	1 oz	105	9	77.1
Cheese, cheddar	1 oz	115	9.4	73.6
Cottage cheese, regular	1 cup	232	10	38.8
Cheese, cottage, low fat (1%)	1 cup	164	2.3	12.6
Cheese, Swiss	1 oz	105	8	68.6
Egg, whole, hard boiled	1	75	5	60
Egg yolk	from 1 egg	60	5.1	76.5
Ice cream	1 cup	264	14.6	49.8
Milkshake, vanilla	12 oz	380	10.3	24.3

Food Items[1]	Amount of Food Items (cooked or prepared)	Total Calories	Fats (g)	% Calories from Fat
Milk, lowfat 1%	1 cup	102	2.6	22.9
Milk, lowfat 2%	1 cup	120	4.7	35.3
Milk, whole	1 cup	150	8.2	49.2
Milk, regular chocolate	1 cup	208	8.5	36.7
Yogurt, regular, plain	1 cup	139	7.4	47.9
Yogurt, fruit flavored	1 cup	253	4.0	14.2
BREADS/CEREALS				
Biscuits	1 each	104	5.1	44.1
Bread, cracked wheat	1 slice	65	1	13.8
Bread, mixed grain	1 slice	65	1	13.8
Bread, oatmeal	1 slice	65	1	13.8
Bread, raisin	1 slice	65	1	13.8
Bread, whole wheat	1 slice	70	1	12.9
English muffin	1 each	140	1.0	6.4
Granola, Nature Valley	1 oz	125	5	36
MISCELLANEOUS				
Avocado	1 medium	306	30	88.2
Butter	1 tbsp	102	11.3	99
Cheesecake	1 slice	256	18	63.3
Cookies, chocolate chip	2 each	160	8	45
Doughnut, plain cake type	1	198	10.8	49.1
Margarine	1 tbsp	102	11.3	99
Mayonnaise	1 tbsp	100	11.2	100
Mixed nuts, dry roasted	1 oz	170	5	11.8
Peanut butter	1 tbsp	95	8	75.8

Food Items[1]	Amount of Food Items (cooked or prepared)	Total Calories	Fats (g)	% Calories from Fat
Peanuts, oil roasted	1 oz	165	8	43.6
Pecans, roasted	0.25 cup	188	19.6	93.8
Salad dressing, Italian	1 tbsp	69	7.1	92.6
Sunflower seeds, dried	1 oz	161	14	78.3
Tofu	0.5 cup	183	11	54.1

[1]Information for most fruits and vegetables is not provided since the contribution from fat is typically < 1% of the energy.

Appendix 3
Protein Content of Selected Foods

Food Items[1]	Amount of Food Item (cooked or prepared)	Total Calories	Protein (grams)	% Calories from Protein
BEEF				
Hamburger, lean ground beef, broiled	4 oz	307	28	36.5
Roast Beef	4 oz	420	25.3	24.0
Steak, sirloin broiled	4 oz	320	30.7	38.4
LAMB				
Lamb Chop, loin broiled	4 oz	336	31.4	37.4
Lamb Rib roasted	4 oz	420	24	22.9
PORK				
Bacon, regular	3 strips	110	6	21.8
Bacon, Canadian style	2 slices	85	11	51.8
Bologna	2 slices	180	7	15.6
Ham, roasted	4 oz	273	24	35.2
Hot Dog	1 each	145	5	13.8
Luncheon Meat	2 slices	140	5	14.3

Food Items[1]	Amount of Food Item (cooked or prepared)	Total Calories	Protein (grams)	% Calories from Protein
Pork chop, broiled	4 oz	355	31	34.9
Salami	2 slices	145	8	22.1
POULTRY				
Chicken, breast roasted w/o skin	4 oz	187	36	77.0
Turkey, light meat	4 oz	180	33.3	74.0
Turkey, dark meat	4 oz	213	32	60.1
FISH AND SHELLFISH				
Fish Sticks	1 each	70	6	34.3
Flounder, baked	4 oz	160	21.3	53.3
Halibut,broiled	4 oz	187	26.7	57.1
Oysters, raw	1 cup	160	20	50.0
Salmon, canned	4 oz	160	22.7	56.8
Sardines, canned	4 oz	233	26.7	45.8
Shrimp, canned	4 oz	133	28	84.2
Tuna, water packed	4 oz	180	40	88.9
Tuna, oil packed	4 oz	220	32	58.2
DAIRY PRODUCTS				
Buttermilk	1 cup	100	8	32.0
Cheese, American	1 oz	105	6	22.9
Cheese, cheddar	1 oz	115	7	24.3
Cottage cheese, regular	1 cup	232	28.1	48.4
Cheese, cottage, low fat (1%)	1 cup	164	28	68.3
Cheese, Swiss	1 oz	95	7	29.5
Egg, whole, hard boiled	1	75	6	32.0

Food Items[1]	Amount of Food Item (cooked or prepared)	Total Calories	Protein (grams)	% Calories from Protein
Egg white	from 1 egg	15	3.8	100
Egg yolk	from 1 egg	60	3	20.0
Instant breakfast	1 pkt	130	7	21.5
Ice cream	1 cup	264	4.6	7.0
Ice milk	1 cup	184	5	11.0
Milkshake, vanilla	12 oz	380	13.2	13.8
Milk, skim	1 cup	85	8.0	37.6
Milk, lowfat 1%	1 cup	100	8	32.0
Milk, lowfat 2%	1 cup	120	8	26.7
Milk, whole	1 cup	150	8	21.3
Milk, regular chocolate	1 cup	208	8	15.4
Yogurt, low fat fruit flavored	8 oz container	230	10	17.4
Yogurt, low fat, plain	8 oz container	145	12	33.1
Yogurt, nonfat plain	8oz container	125	13	41.6

BEANS/ LENTILS/ DRIED PEAS

Baked beans, canned	1 cup	236	12	20.3
Black beans	1 cup	225	15	26.7
Chickpeas	1 cup	270	15	22.2
Green peas	1 cup	115	8	27.8
Kidney beans	1 cup	230	15	26.1
Lentils	1 cup	215	16	29.8
Lima beans	1 cup	260	16	24.6
Navy beans	1 cup	225	15	26.7
Pinto beans	1 cup	265	15	22.6

Food Items[1]	Amount of Food Item (cooked or prepared)	Total Calories	Protein (grams)	% Calories from Protein
Refried beans	1 cup	295	18	24.4
Tofu	1/2 cup	183	19.9	43.6
BREADS AND GRAINS				
Bagel	1 each	200	7	14.0
Biscuits	1 each	95	2	8.4
Bread, cracked wheat	1 slice	65	2	12.3
Bread, mixed grain	1 slice	65	2	12.3
Bread, oatmeal	1 slice	65	2	12.3
Bread, raisin	1 slice	65	2	12.3
Bread, whole wheat	1 slice	70	3	17.1
English muffin	1 each	140	5	14.3
Muffin, Blueberry or Bran	1 each	140	3	8.6
Pancakes, plain	1 each	60	2	13.3
Pita bread, large, white	6.5" round	165	6	14.5
Pasta, egg noodles	1 cup	200	7	14.0
Spaghetti, enriched	1 cup	155	5	12.9
Rice, white	1 cup	225	4	7.1
Rice, brown long grain	1 cup	216	5	9.3
CEREALS				
All Bran	1 oz	70	4	22.9
40% Bran Flakes	1 oz	90	3.6	14.1
Cheerios	1 oz	110	4	14.5
Granola, Nature Valley	1 oz	125	3	9.6
Grape-Nuts	1 oz	100	3	12.0

Food Items[1]	Amount of Food Item (cooked or prepared)	Total Calories	Protein (grams)	% Calories from Protein
Oatmeal, nonfortified	1 cup	145	6	16.6
Raisin Bran	1 oz	90	3	13.3
Shredded Wheat	1 biscuit	83	2.6	12.0
Special K	1 oz	110	6	21.8
Total	1 oz	100	3	12.0
Wheaties	1 oz	100	3	12.0
MISCELLANEOUS				
Peanut butter	1 tbsp	95	5	21.1
Brewers yeast	1 tbsp	25	3	48.0
Sunflower seeds	1 oz	160	6	15.0
Peanuts, oil roasted	1 oz	165	8	19.4
Mixed nuts, dry roasted	1 oz	170	5	11.8

[1]Information for cookies, crackers, cakes, fruits, and vegetables is not provided since the contribution of protein is typically less than 1% of the total energy.

Appendix 4
Energy Expenditure For Various Activities

Activities	kcal/min	kcal/hr
Archery	5	273
Badminton	7	407
Basketball - Half Court	4	256
Basketball - Full Court	7	433
Bowling	4	252
Boxing - Sparring	10	580
Calisthenics, Strenuous	9	540
Canoeing - Leisure	3	185
Canoeing - Racing	7	433
Card Playing	2	105
Carpentry - General	4	218
Carpet Sweeping	3	189
Climbing Hills - No Load	8	508
Climbing Hills - Loaded 5 Kg	9	546
Climbing Hills - Loaded 10 Kg	10	588
Climbing Hills - Loaded 20 Kg	11	630

Activities	kcal/min	kcal/hr
Cycling - 5 To 10 MPH	6	336
Cycling - 10 To 15 MPH	8	504
Cycling - 15 To 20 MPH	11	672
Cycling - Racing	14	848
Dancing - Rock	5	273
Digging Trenches	10	609
Dips - 20 per minute	4	261
Eating	2	97
Electrical Work	4	244
Fishing	4	260
Football	9	546
Gardening - Raking	4	227
Gardening - Planting By Hand	8	462
Gardening - Hedging	5	323
Gardening - Mowing By Hand	8	462
Gardening - Digging	9	529
Golf - 2some	6	340
Golf - 4some	4	248
Grocery Shopping	4	252
Handball	11	659
Judo/karate	14	819
Lying At Ease	2	92
Mopping Floor	4	252
Obstacle Course	10	600

Activities	kcal/min	kcal/hr
Outdoor Work - Sawing By Hand	8	504
Outdoor Work - Carrying Logs	13	756
Outdoor Work - Sawing By Power	5	315
Outdoor Work - Barking Trees	8	504
Outdoor Work - Weeding	5	302
Outdoor Work - Chopping Wood	21	1,260
Painting Inside	2	143
Painting Outside	5	323
Playing Ping Pong	5	286
Playing Pool	3	176
Push-Ups- 20 per minute	6	341
Reading	2	105
Rockclimbing	7	420
Roller Blading - Moderate	6	349
Roller Blading - Vigorous	11	638
Rowing - 15 To 20 Strokes/min	9	546
Rowing - 20 To 25 Strokes/min	12	714
Rowing - 25 To 30 Strokes/min	14	848
Rowing - 30 To 35 Strokes/min	16	937
Rowing - 35 To 40 Strokes/min	20	1,172
Rugby/Soccer	9	554
Run - 5.5 Min Per Mile	19	1,134
Run - 6 Min Per Mile	18	1,058
Run - 7 Min Per Mile	16	958

Activities	kcal/min	kcal/hr
Run - 8 Min Per Mile	14	811
Run - 9 Min Per Mile	12	714
Run - 10 Min Per Mile	11	651
Run - 11 Min Per Mile	9	567
Scraping Paint	4	265
Scrubbing Floors	8	462
Scuba Diving, Leisurely	14	865
Scuba Diving, Vigorous	19	1,159
Sit-Ups - 20 per minute	5	330
Sitting in the Cold	3	180
Sitting Quietly	1	88
Skiing, Downhill - Moderate Speed	8	500
Skiing, Downhill - Leisurely (M)	7	420
Skiing, Crosscountry - Uphill	19	1,151
Skiing, Crosscountry - Walking	10	601
Skipping Rope	12	739
Sleeping/napping	1	42
Snowshoeing - Soft Snow	12	697
Squash - Doubles	7	445
Squash - Singles	15	890
Stairclimbing - Slow	9	538
Stairclimbing - Moderate	11	659
Stairclimbing - Fast	15	874
Standing Quietly	2	109

Activities	kcal/min	kcal/hr
Swimming - Treading Fast	12	714
Swimming - Treading Slow	4	260
Swimming - Breaststroke	11	680
Swimming - Backstroke	12	710
Swimming - Crawl Fast	14	840
Swimming - Side Stroke	9	512
Swimming - Crawl Slow	9	538
Tennis, Singles	8	458
Tennis, Doubles	6	336
Video Games, Watching	2	105
Volleyball	4	210
Walking with 70 lb pack - 3 MPH at 2.5% grade	7	439
Washing Dishes	3	155
Watching TV/movies	1	88
Weight/Circuit Training - Nautilus	11	630
Writing/Drawing	2	122

Note: The energy expenditure values in this appendix are for a 70 Kg (155 lb) man and are intended to provide you with an estimate. Your values may be lower or higher depending on your body weight.

Appendix 5
Good Food Sources of Vitamins

Nutrient	Vitamin Food Sources	Nutrient Content in Selected Food
Vitamin A	green and yellow fruits and vegetables, milk, milk products, fish liver oil, liver	beef liver broiled, 4 oz. 40,900 IU sweet potato baked, 1 med 24,880 IU carrots raw, 1 med. 20,250 IU spinach cooked, 1 cup 14,740 IU apricots dried, 7 halves 2,350 IU
Vitamin D	egg yolks, organ meats, bone meal, fortified milk, salmon, sunlight	salmon/tuna canned, 4 oz. 568 IU sardines canned, 4 oz. 340 IU milk 2%, 1 cup 100 IU chicken liver, 4 oz. 60 IU egg yolk, 1 each 25 IU
Vitamin E	seed oils, dark green vegetables, eggs, nuts, liver, organ meats, wheat germ, milk fat, desiccated liver	wheat germ oil, 1 **table spoon (tbsp)** 52 IU sunflower oil, 1 tbsp 13 IU milk nonfat, 1 cup 11.3 IU avocado Florida, 1 whole 6 IU peas cooked, 1 cup 3.4 IU salmon broiled, 4 oz. 2.5 IU

Nutrient	Vitamin Food Sources	Nutrient Content in Selected Food
Vitamin K	green and/or leafy vegetables	parsley, 10 sprigs 70 µg spinach raw chopped, 1 cup 192.5 µg kale cooked, 1 cup 975 µg broccoli cooked, 1 cup 310 µg brussels sprouts cooked, 1 cup 341 µg
Vitamin B$_1$ Thiamin	blackstrap molasses, brewer's yeast, whole grains, legumes, pork, nuts, organ meats, wheat germ	brewers yeast, 2 tbsp 1.25 mg sunflower seeds, 2 tbsp 1.3 mg pork chop broiled, 4 oz. 1.1 mg pecans, 2 tbsp 0.5 mg black beans cooked, 1 cup 0.4 mg brown rice cooked, 1 cup 0.2 mg
Vitamin B$_2$ Riboflavin	milk and dairy products, green leafy vegetables, black-strap molasses, nuts, organ meats, whole grains	beef liver broiled, 4 oz. 3.5 mg corn grits cooked, 1 cup 2.0 mg yogurt nonfat, 1 cup 0.5 mg almonds, 2 tbsp 0.4 mg spinach cooked, 1 cup 0.4 mg
Vitamin B$_3$ Niacin	brewer's yeast, seafood, lean meats, milk, milk products, poultry, desiccated liver	beef liver broiled, 4 oz. 12 mg chicken breast roasted, 4 oz. 15.7 mg hamburger broiled, 4 oz. 5.5 mg peanut butter, 2 tbsp 4.4 mg mushrooms raw, 1 cup 2.9 mg tomato juice, 1 cup 1.6 mg
Pantothenic Acid	Present in all plant and animal foods, brewer's yeast, legumes, organ meats, salmon, wheat germ, whole grains	beef liver broiled, 4 oz. 6.7 mg corn cooked, 1 cup 1.4 mg salmon baked, 4 oz. 1.3 mg milk 2%, 1 cup 0.8 mg wheat germ toasted, 2 tbsp 0.6 mg orange juice fresh, 1 cup 0.4 mg

Nutrient	Vitamin Food Sources	Nutrient Content in Selected Food
Vitamin B$_6$	blackstrap molasses, brewer's yeast, meat, organ meats, poultry, wheat germ, whole grains, and yeast	beef liver, 4 oz. 1.6 mg banana, 1 med 0.7 mg sunflower seeds, 2 tbsp 0.5 mg brussels sprouts cooked, 1 cup 0.3 mg brown rice, 1 cup 0.3 mg wheat germ toasted, 2 tbsp 0.3 mg prunes dried, 10 each 0.2 mg
Vitamin B$_{12}$	cheese, fish, milk, milk products, organ meats, shellfish and eggs	beef liver broiled, 4 oz. 127 μg tuna canned, 4 oz. 3.7 μg hamburger broiled, 4 oz. 2.8 μg cottage cheese creamed, 1 cup 1.3 μg milk lowfat, 1 cup 0.9 μg yogurt nonfat, 1 cup 0.6 μg egg cooked, 1 med 0.6 μg
Biotin	legumes, whole grains, organ meats, and eggs	brewer's yeast, 2 tbsp 120 μg beef liver, 4 oz. 112 μg wheat germ, 2 tbsp 14 μg peanut butter, 2tbsp 12 μg egg cooked, 1 med 12 μg
Folic acid folacin	dark green leafy vegetables, milk, milk products, organ meats, oysters, salmon, whole grains	brewer's yeast, 2 tbsp 626 μg spinach steamed, 1 cup 448 μg beef liver broiled, 4 oz. 249 μg orange juice, 1 cup 109 μg wheat germ toasted, 2 tbsp 100 μg broccoli cooked, 1 cup 78 μg romaine lettuce, 1 cup 76 μg cottage cheese creamed, 1 cup 26 μg egg hardboiled, 1 med 24 μg
Vitamin C Ascorbate	citrus fruits, other fruits and vegetables	cantaloupe, 1/2 melon 113 mg grapefruit, 1 med 100 mg broccoli cooked, 1 cup 97 mg peppers green, 1 med 95 mg strawberries, 1 cup 90 mg orange, 1 med 70 mg watermelon, 1 slice, 46 mg white potato baked no skin, 1 med 26 mg sweet potato baked, 1 med 28 mg

Appendix 6
Good Food Sources
of Minerals

Nutrient	Food Sources of Minerals	Nutrient Content in Selected Food
Boron	fruits, leafy vegetables, nuts, lentils, bean and legumes	pear, 1 med 420 µg dates, 5 each 400 µg apple, 1 med 153 µg peach, 1 med 119 µg peanuts, 2 tbsp 100 µg carrot, 1 med 78 µg
Calcium	milk, cheese, yogurt, green leafy vegetables, beans and legumes	Swiss cheese, 4 oz. 520 mg lowfat milk, 1 cup 297 mg spinach cooked, 1 cup 245 mg black beans cooked, 1 cup 140 mg broccoli cooked, 1 cup 71 mg
Chromium	whole grains, cheese, brewer's yeast and beer	broccoli steamed, 1 cup 22 µg ham cooked, 4 oz. 4.8 µg turkey breast baked, 4 oz. 2.3 µg green beans cooked, 1 cup 2.2 µg banana, 1 med 1 µg beer, 12 oz. 0.17 to 20 µg

Nutrient	Food Sources of Minerals	Nutrient Content in Selected Food
Copper	nuts, organ meats, whole grain cereal, and legumes, dried fruit	beef liver broiled, 4 oz. 3.2 mg black-eyed peas cooked, 1 cup 1.4 mg cashews, 2 tbsp 0.8 mg blackstrap molasses, 2 tbsp 0.6 mg
Iron	meat, liver, blackstrap molasses, dark green vegetables, enriched grains, legumes	beef liver broiled, 4 oz. 7.0 mg blackstrap molasses, 2 tbsp 5.0 mg hamburger broiled, 4 oz. 2.7 mg oatmeal, cooked, 1 cup 1.6 mg raisins, 1/2 cup 1.5 mg apricots dried, 7 halves 1 mg
Magnesium	nuts, wheat germ, whole grains, seafood, fruits, and green leafy vegetables	tofu firm, 1 cup 236 mg Swiss chard cooked, 1 cup 150 mg wheat germ toasted, 2 tbsp 90 mg cashews roasted, 2 tbsp 89 mg brown rice, 1 cup 86 mg potato baked with skin, 1 med 55 mg green peas cooked, 1 cup 46 mg
Manganese	nuts, legumes, whole grain cereals	wheat germ toasted, 2 tbsp 5.7 mg brown rice cooked, 1 cup 2.1 mg oatmeal cooked, 1 cup 1.4 mg
Phosphorous	milk, milk products, meats, poultry, fish, legumes and nuts	lentils cooked, 1 cup 356 mg wheat germ toasted, 2 tbsp 325mg salmon canned, 4 oz. 325 mg milk 2%, 1 cup 232 mg almonds, 2 tbsp 184 mg oatmeal cooked, 1 cup 178 mg
Potassium	fruits such as bananas, watermelon, oranges and dates, bran cereals and vegetables,	baked potato w/ skin, 1 med 844 mg lima beans cooked, 1 cup 694 mg watermelon, 1 slice 600 mg banana, 1 med 569 mg cantaloupe 1/2 med 502 mg apricots dried, 8 halves 490 mg oranges, 1 med 311 mg

Nutrient	Food Sources of Minerals	Nutrient Content in Selected Food
Selenium	meats, seafood and cereals	Brazil nuts, 2 tbsp 380 µg salmon baked, 4 oz. 93 µg hamburger broiled, 4 oz. 29 µg wheat germ toasted, 2 tbsp 28 µg blackstrap molasses, 2 tbsp 25 µg egg boiled, 1 each 12 µg
Sodium	widely present in all foods (especially processed foods) except fruit	table salt cottage cheese 2%, 1 cup 918 mg cheddar cheese, 2 oz. 352 mg ice cream, 1 cup 166 mg milk 2%, 1 cup 120 mg
Zinc	animal and seafood, eggs and dairy products, whole grain breads, cereals, legumes, peanuts	oysters, Eastern, 1 cup 226 mg hamburger broiled, 4 oz. 6.2 mg turkey dark meat baked, 4 oz. 5 mg wheat germ toasted, 2 tbsp 4.7 mg pecans, 2 tbsp 1.6 mg peanut butter, 2 tbsp 1.4 mg salmon baked, 4 oz. 0.5 mg

Appendix 7
Sample High Carbohydrate Menus

Sample Day One

BREAKFAST		LUNCH	
Orange juice	1 cup	Turkey sandwich	
Hard cooked eggs	2 eggs	Turkey breast sliced	4 oz
Whole wheat toasts	2 each	Whole wheat bread	2 slices
Margarine	1 pat	Lettuce, iceberg	1/4 cup
Blueberry muffin	1 each	Tomato	1/2
Banana	1 each	Mustard	1 tsp
Coffee w/milk & sugar	1 cup	Miracle whip	1 Tbsp
MORNING SNACK		Carrot	2 med
Bagel	1 each	Chocolate milk, low fat	1 cup
w/ jam & peanut butter	1 Tbsp ea	**AFTERNOON SNACK**	
Apple	1 each	Orange juice	1 cup
Instant breakfast	1 packet	Granola bar - Oats n honey	1 bar
w/ skim milk	1 cup		

DINNER		DINNER continued	
Spaghetti, cooked	2 cups	Carrots, grated	1/4 cup
Spaghetti sauce w/mush-rooms	1/2 cup	Low fat salad dressing	2 Tbsp
Parmesan cheese	1 Tbsp	Hot fudge sundae	1 serving
French bread w/	1/4 loaf	Orange juice	1 cup
Garlic butter	2 pats	**BEDTIME SNACK**	
Salad w/		Ovaltine (malt flavored)	1 cup
Lettuce	1/2 cup	Oatmeal & raisin cookies	4 each
Tomato	1 each		
Cucumber	1/2 cup		

Macronutrient Analysis of Day One

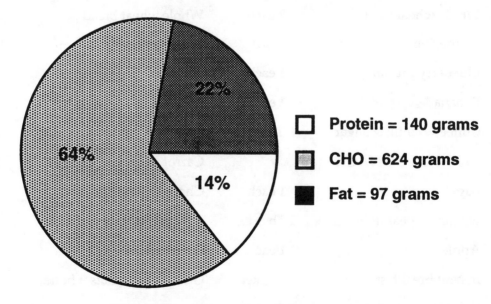

Protein = 140 grams

CHO = 624 grams

Fat = 97 grams

Total Energy = 3,850 kcal

Sample High Carbohydrate Menus

Sample Day Two

BREAKFAST

Cranberry juice	1 cup
Pancakes	3 each
Maple syrup-lite	3 Tbsp
Butter	2 pats
Milk, skim	1 cup
Apple	1 each
Coffee (w/ milk & sugar)	1 cup

MORNING SNACK

Bran muffin	1 each
Banana	1 each
Low fat chocolate milk	1 cup

LUNCH

Tuna salad sandwich	
Tuna packed in water	1oz
Celery, diced	1/8 cup
Miracle whip	2 Tbsp
Pumpernickel bread	2 slices
Lettuce, iceberg	1/8 cup
Tomato	1/2 each
Mustard	1 tsp
Yogurt, low fat -fruit flavored	1 cup
Orange juice	2 cups

AFTERNOON SNACK

Apple juice	12 oz can
Milky way bar	1 bar

DINNER

Roasted chicken breast w/ out skin	1 breast
Steamed vegetable	
Broccoli	1/3 cup
Carrots	1/3 cup
Cauliflower	1/3 cup
Baked potato	1 each
Sour cream	2 Tbsp
Whole wheat dinner rolls	2 rolls
Butter/ margarine	1 pat
Brownies w/ nuts	2 each
Strawberries	1 cup
Orange juice	1 cup

BEDTIME SNACK

Ovaltine malt flavor	1 cup
Whole wheat crackers	3 each
Cheddar cheese	0.5 oz

Macronutrient Analysis of Day Two

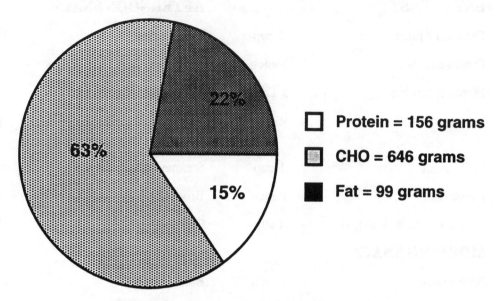

22%

63%

15%

Protein = 156 grams

CHO = 646 grams

Fat = 99 grams

Total Energy = 3,990 kcal

Sample Day Three

BREAKFAST		MORNING SNACK	
Apple juice	1 cup	Banana	1 each
Wheaties	1 bowl	Orange juice	1 cup
Milk, skim	1 cup	**LUNCH**	
Whole wheat toasts	2 each	McDLT sandwich	1 each
Peanut butter	1 Tbsp	Apple	1 each
Grape jelly	1 Tbsp	Orange juice	1 cup
Coffee (w/ milk & sugar)	1 cup		

AFTERNOON SNACK		DINNER continued	
Apple juice	12 oz can	Carrots, grated or chopped	1/4 cup
Fruit bar - oat bran & nuts	1 each	Broccoli	1/3 cup
DINNER		Non fat salad dressing	2 Tbsp
Pizza- combination supreme- medium	6 slices	Peach cobbler	1 serving
Salad w/		Orange juice	1 cup
Lettuce	1/4 cup	**BEDTIME SNACK**	
Tomato	1 each	Milk, skim	1 cup
Cauliflower	1/4 cup	Chocolate chip cookies	4 each

Macronutrient Analysis of Day Three

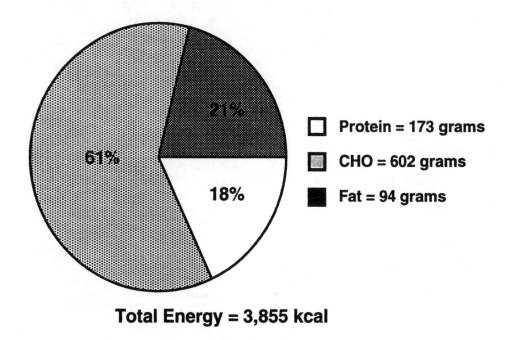

21%

61%

18%

☐ Protein = 173 grams

▨ CHO = 602 grams

■ Fat = 94 grams

Total Energy = 3,855 kcal

Appendix 8
US Navy Special Warfare
10 Commandments Of
Nutrition

1. Don't believe anything you read about nutrition written by someone trying to sell you something.

2. Read the labels on food products. Total calories and weights of carbohydrate (CHO), protein, and fat per serving are usually provided.

3. Most Americans need no supplemental vitamins, but use the inexpensive "one-a-day" type if you want to increase your vitamin intake. Megadose quantities of costly wonder-vitamins serve mainly to increase the vitamin content of your body waste products.

4. Don't take protein and amino acid supplements. One gram of protein per pound of body weight per day is the maximum recommended protein intake, even for weight training and body building. Most non-vegetarian athletes take in more than this in their normal diet

5. Limit fat intake to less than 30% of total calories (1 gram of fat = 9 calories). Items to watch are red meat, peanuts, solid dairy products, and french-fried anything.

6. For specific endurance events such as prolonged missions, long cold dives, or triathalons, CHO load with 1500 extra CHO calories a day for 3 days before the event and decrease fat and protein intake. Cut back on your training schedule and avoid stressful cold exposures during this time.

7. For prolonged intense aerobic training schedules (BUD/s or triathalon training), take in enough extra CHO calories to maintain your desired weight. The best sources are pasta, fruits, breads, potatoes, and rice.

8. Eat fresh fruits, fresh vegetables, and high-fiber cereal products every day.

9. Short-term weight reduction diets are generally useless and occasionally dangerous. Lasting weight modification is accomplished only with long-term changes in your eating and exercise habits.

10. The most common nutrition problem in this country is too much nutrition. Don't eat when you're not hungry and stop eating as soon as you've had enough, not when your plate is empty.

Full Mission Profile, January 1992
Compliments of CAPT Frank Butler